The Psychology of Coming Out

"In *The Psychology of Coming Out*, Professor Rusi Jaspal, a leading figure in LGBTQ+ scholarship, has produced what I have no doubt is a landmark contribution and an essential read for anyone seeking to understand the deeply personal, yet profoundly social, journey of coming out.

Through compelling case studies and thematic analyses, Professor Jaspal gives voice to a diverse range of LGB coming out experiences across varied contexts, all illuminated with care, dignity, and scholarly depth.

This book is not only an important scholarly investigation into identity processes associated with coming out, it is also a compassionately written window into the wider psychological journey of LGB individuals and as such will be of great relevance to clinicians, educators, EDI professionals, family members, and policymakers and is a call to action for society to create environments where LGB individuals can thrive and be supported. A true milestone in LGBTQ+ Psychology."

—Professor Marco Cinnirella, *Professor of Applied Social Psychology, Royal Holloway, University of London, UK*

"Rusi Jaspal's *The Psychology of Coming Out: Lesbian, Gay, and Bisexual Identities* offers a thought-provoking and nuanced exploration of the psychological dimensions of coming out, with a particular emphasis on global and cross-cultural contexts.

Drawing on extensive research, Jaspal delves into the lived experiences of disclosing one's sexual identity, examining how this pivotal act influences personal cognition, interpersonal relationships, and the broader construction and defense of identity. He carefully considers both the benefits and challenges associated with coming out, providing a comprehensive analysis that bridges individual experience with sociocultural frameworks.

This book is a valuable resource for university students at all levels—undergraduate and graduate alike—as well as for researchers interested in the theoretical and methodological underpinnings of coming out processes."

—Professor Christian Grov, *Distinguished Professor of Public Health, CUNY Graduate School of Public Health and Health Policy, New York, USA*

"This book presents a comprehensive and very clearly expressed account of theory, process, and lived experience of "coming out" for lesbian, gay, and bisexual (LGB) people. It incorporates a detailed critique of the vast research on the topic, as well as presenting a new and integrated way to think about coming out as both an event and as a continued life-long process. Especially interesting is the inclusion of new data on the lived experience of coming out and how these data may help us to understand individuals' experiences from the words of the individuals themselves. These data also highlight the many complexities associated with coming out for LGB people within heteronormative societies. This book is an important read for all, and especially for anyone working in the educational, health, and helping professions."

—Dr Claire Bloxsom, *UKCP Registered Integrative Psychotherapist, BPS Chartered Psychologist, Nottingham, UK*

"*The Psychology of Coming Out* is a landmark contribution to our understanding of lesbian, gay, and bisexual identities. Rusi Jaspal offers a compelling, theory-informed analysis of the psychological processes involved in coming out, drawing on rich empirical data and global perspectives. This book challenges assumptions about coming out, highlights the complexity of the process and experience of coming out, and culminates in a novel framework that will no doubt prove invaluable for further research and interventions aimed at supporting LGB individuals in diverse contexts. It is essential reading for scholars, practitioners, and students alike."

—Professor David M. Frost, *Professor of Social Psychology, University College London, London, UK*

Rusi Jaspal

The Psychology of Coming Out

Lesbian, Gay, and Bisexual Identities

palgrave
macmillan

Rusi Jaspal
Vice-Chancellor's Office
University of Brighton
Brighton, UK

ISBN 978-3-032-02598-2 ISBN 978-3-032-02599-9 (eBook)
https://doi.org/10.1007/978-3-032-02599-9

This Palgrave Macmillan imprint is published by the registered company Springer Nature Switzerland AG.
The registered company address is: Gewerbestrasse 11, 6330 Cham, Switzerland

This book is dedicated to the memory of my mother A. D. Jaspal (1956–2021) whose response to my coming out was inspiring.

Acknowledgements

This book is the product of many stimulating conversations over the years with hundreds of students, colleagues, and, most importantly, lesbian, gay, and bisexual people about coming out. Our discussions made me realize that a book on the realities of coming out in the twenty-first century was much needed.

I am grateful my former and present PhD students Moubadda Assi, Anthony Gifford, Dr. Ismael Maatouk, and Razina Mamadbai, all of whom have tackled questions of sexuality and identity in their own research, from their own perspectives, and in novel contexts. Their projects demonstrate cultural differences in coming out but also the global relevance of coming out regardless of these differences.

Finally, I am grateful to my family for their unwavering support as I worked on this and other books.

Competing Interests The author has no competing interests to declare that are relevant to the content of this manuscript.

Contents

List of Figures

List of Tables

1

The Psychology of Coming Out: An Introduction

The purpose of this book is to examine the psychological aspects of coming out as lesbian, gay, or bisexual (LGB). There is a particular focus upon the effects of coming out for identity processes. Put simply, the aim is to shed light on what happens to the identity of the LGB person when they come out to people who matter to them. The book explores what we already know about the psychology of coming out based on previous studies and what can be gleaned from the first-hand accounts of LGB people who have come out to somebody significant.

Many studies have examined differences between subgroups of LGB people in their experiences of coming out, with mixed findings (e.g., Anderson-Carpenter, 2022; Kuyper & Vanwesenbeeck, 2011; Maatouk & Jaspal, 2023; Pistella et al., 2020; Rehman et al., 2020; White & Stephenson, 2013). This is not the aim of this book. Rather, this book explores what the experience of telling somebody significant that one is LGB feels like, how it informs people's thinking and their relationships with their significant others, and, crucially, how coming out shapes the construction, development, and defense of identity. It examines the shared aspects of experience among LGB people with an emphasis on what happens to identity processes, rather than the content of identity

R. Jaspal, *The Psychology of Coming Out*,
https://doi.org/10.1007/978-3-032-02599-9_1

itself. The findings of the studies reported in this book contribute to the development of a theoretical framework in which the antecedents, consequences, and experiences of coming out can be collectively examined. The framework outlined in the final chapter of this book should be used to inform interventions for supporting LGB people as they contemplate coming out and when they actually do so.

The Complexities of Coming Out

Coming out is a vast topic. Over the life course, LGB people may come out to many different groups and individuals. They come out repeatedly as they encounter novel contexts and situations. They may even need to come out to the same group or individual more than once. LGB people vary in the extent to which they come out to each group or individual, with some people coming to know more about their sexuality than others. For many LGB people, coming out to their family (and especially to their parents) is especially significant. Indeed, most but not all respondents whose accounts are reproduced in this book focused on their experiences of coming out to their parents and immediate family members when asked to reflect upon a significant coming out experience.

No single coming out experience is the same. Coming out means different things to different people and is experienced in different ways. Many factors shape the experience of coming out—personality, culture, the availability of social support, the legal status of LGB people, and even the availability of identity categories, such as "lesbian," "gay," and "bisexual," in one's culture.

Coming out is not just about telling another person that one is LGB. It is also about the broader changes that the experience of self-disclosure brings about in the coming-out individual's own identity and in their relationships with others. Indeed, coming out is experienced differently because the identity of every coming-out individual is unique. Three case studies can be used to exemplify the diverse experiences of LGB people in relation to coming out.

Santiago

Santiago is a 24-year-old gay man living in Cali, Colombia. He has always known he is gay but, given his conservative Evangelical upbringing, also knows that his parents would never accept his sexuality. He has always kept his sexuality a secret, although he is aware that his parents and siblings suspect that he is gay.

His father often makes disparaging comments about gay people, adding that he would disown a family member—including his own children—if they ever came out as gay. Santiago views this as a personal warning to him. Santiago's father often obliges him to accompany him to Church where the pastor regularly delivers religious sermons condemning homosexuality. These religious diatribes against homosexuality, which Santiago knows influence his father's views, have led him to question his self-worth and, more recently, his own Christian faith. Although less religious than his father, Santiago's mother also contributes to his feelings of guilt and shame in relation to his sexuality—she often makes negative remarks about his hairstyle, appearance, and demeanor, implying that they are "girly." His brothers never make comments about homosexuality but they do avoid talking about girls whenever he is around. This contributes to Santiago's fears that his family all know that he is gay. He worries that they may be talking about this among themselves and thinking all sorts of negative thoughts about him. Santiago is confused about his feelings regarding his family's behavior—on the one hand, he prefers to avoid confrontation but, on the other hand, feels that he is living a lie. Neighbors sometimes question why he—a handsome young man—has never had a girlfriend. All these comments make Santiago—and his family, he knows—feel immensely uncomfortable. He is especially concerned that his sexuality may be involuntarily disclosed. Together, these experiences are making him feel anxious and depressed.

Santiago previously saw no way out of this difficult situation but now has several sources of support. Santiago has four close female friends, all of whom know he is gay. He confides in them and feels that he can be himself when he is with them. However, he sometimes feels that he has to explain himself to them when, for instance, they question why he does not just tell his parents that he is gay. At times he feels judged for being inauthentic. A year ago, his life changed significantly—he began to communicate with Adam, who lives in Europe, on a social networking platform. His relationship with Adam has given him much more confidence. He had previously felt that he was unworthy of love and that he would never get into a relationship with anyone else, not least a man. Things have changed—Santiago and Adam hope to live together one day. However, their relationship is not without its challenges. In order to meet Adam when he visits Colombia, Santiago has to invent a pretext for leaving his home. He has become accustomed to lying to his family. His relationship with Adam is important to him but his family situation is having an impact on their relationship. Adam is growing impatient about the future, but Santiago sees no way of coming out to his family and therefore living openly with Adam. He fantasizes about living secretly with Adam without his parents ever finding out. He is acutely aware that this is unfeasible but the prospect of coming out to his family fills him with dread. Even with Adam, he avoids talking about coming out.

Rahul

Rahul is a 39-year-old bisexual man living in London, United Kingdom. He is British and of South Asian descent. Growing up in a conservative Indian family, Rahul had felt fearful about coming out as bisexual and believed that his parents would never understand or accept his sexuality.

Rahul had had several girlfriends but, when he was 16, started a romantic relationship with an older man. His mother found a love letter that he had written to his partner and discovered that he was in a homosexual relationship. For weeks, his mother was cold toward him but he did not understand why until he finally confronted her about her aloof behavior. An argument ensued between them in which Rahul's mother accused him of being immoral and promiscuous without explicitly mentioning his sexuality. When he told her he was bisexual, she did not appear to understand what this meant. She kept contradicting him, reminding him that he had had several girlfriends and that he was not gay. When Rahul retorted that he was bisexual, his mother began to weep, stating that, while she did not accept his sexuality, she still loved him as he was her son. Rahul felt torn—on the one hand, he felt a sense of relief that he no longer needed to lie but, on the other hand, he felt extremely guilty about how this situation had made his mother feel. He felt that he had failed her. She too implied this, stating that she had done all she could as a mother and questioned where she had "gone wrong."

To assuage his mother's concerns, Rahul assured her that his same-sex relationship was just an experiment—a phase—and that he was really heterosexual. Deep down, he knew that this was just a pretense, but this half-truth was preferable to the pain that he felt he was causing his mother. Rahul had tried to come out but now felt that this had to be undone. He and his mother never discussed his sexuality again and, as a proponent of arranged marriage, his mother regularly brought marriage proposals to his attention, all of which he immediately rejected. She became suspicious when he brought home male friends, clearly suspecting that Rahul might be romantically involved with them. All this caused a significant rift in their relationship which led him to leave home when he completed his university education. These days, their occasional conversations over the telephone are curt and superficial. Rahul's mother occasionally makes disparaging comments about homosexuality and people that she suspects of being gay. His mother's complete denial of his sexuality sometimes makes Rahul question whether his coming out experience ever actually took place. Rahul fears that the topic of his sexuality may be broached and does not wish to feel the guilt and shame that his first coming out experience induced. He misses his mother and wishes that they could reconcile their relationship. He does not know how to do this.

Sharon

Sharon is an 18-year-old lesbian woman living in Flagstaff, Arizona, United States. She lives with her parents who are relatively liberal and with whom she has always had a close relationship.

When Sharon was 14, she realized that she was attracted to girls in her class and was not interested in the attention she received from boys. She began to think that she might be a lesbian and, some months later, decided to confide in her parents one evening after school. They asked her if she was sure and, while surprised to hear this, were very accepting, reassuring her that they would always be supportive. Sharon felt a great weight off her shoulders, which in turn enabled her to confide in her parents about her feelings and about other aspects of her life—even those unrelated to her sexuality. She felt that coming out as a lesbian had truly strengthened her relationship with her parents.

Although her parents were apparently accepting of her sexuality, they asked her not to share this information with members of their extended family. This made Sharon feel confused—on the one hand, her parents made her feel that she could be herself with them but, on the other hand, they appeared to be asking her to conceal what she now considered to be an important part of her identity. She became resentful toward them and defiantly decided to tell her cousin that she was a lesbian. Her cousin seemed shocked and told her that she did not look like a lesbian. He began to ask her intrusive questions about her sexuality, such as what made her "become" a lesbian, as well as questions about her sexual experiences with women. She felt ridiculed and fetishized—most notably because she believed that her cousin reduced her lesbian identity to sex.

What Sharon finds most uncomfortable is that she cannot be as open about her sexuality with friends and extended family members as she can with her parents. She realizes that she repeatedly has to come out—when she meets new people—and never knows what their reaction will be. Most of her coming out experiences are positive and make her feel confident and positive about herself. Occasionally, her experiences are negative and they chip away at her self-worth. She is selective about whom she tells but, when she encounters a negative reaction, recalls her most positive coming out experience—to her parents.

The three real-life case studies of a gay man, lesbian women, and bisexual man in three distinct socio-cultural contexts illustrate some of the themes that characterize LGB people's coming out experiences and that are discussed in this book: the role of religion and other group memberships (such as the family itself) in self-definition and coming out; the perceived need to conceal one's sexuality and pass as heterosexual to avoid stigma;

mixed messages about one's sexuality; fear of involuntary disclosure of one's sexuality; implicit awareness but silence regarding one's sexuality; emotional distance from loved ones as a result of coming out; self-acceptance; perceived acceptance; a strengthening of bonds with significant others; feeling loved; the role of romantic relationships; repeatedly having to come out; feeling reassured, supported, and empowered to come out to more people; and many others. They also highlight the multitude of emotions that LGB people experience based largely upon the reaction that they encounter from somebody that matters: guilt; shame; fear; anxiety; relief; happiness; hope; disappointment; conflict; and many others. The case studies demonstrate the varying degrees of outness experienced by LGB people. They evidence the inextricable, reciprocal links between interpersonal interactions and cognition, affect, and behavior. How LGB people think about their identity shapes their decision-making regarding coming out, and their interpersonal interactions with others shape how they in turn think about their identity and indeed future decision-making regarding coming out to others. Many of these issues have been examined in previous research and are discussed throughout this book.

Definitions and Clarifications

In this book, the terms "sexuality," "sexual identity," "identity processes," "coming out," "outness," "closetedness," and "significant others" are used. These terms are contentious, used and understood in different ways, and, therefore, must be defined. Additionally, common approaches to measuring outness are outlined.

Sexuality, Sexual Identity, and Identity Processes

The terms "sexual orientation" and "sexuality" are used interchangeably to refer to "a trait that predisposes an individual to experience sexual attraction to people of the same sex (gay [or lesbian]), to people of the opposite sex (heterosexual), or to people of both sexes (bisexual)" (Jaspal, 2019, p. 19). In contrast, sexual identity refers to the individual's own perception of their sexuality as an element of their identity when it has been assimilated and accommodated within the identity structure. Strictly speaking, sexuality becomes an element of identity but for convenience it is referred to as "sexual identity" throughout this book. Identity processes, which are discussed in greater detail in Chap. 3, refer to changes that occur in relation to the processes of assimilation-accommodation and evaluation. These include changes to the content of identity, to the hierarchical organization of identity elements, or to the value of identity elements (Breakwell, 1986).

Coming Out, Outness, and Closetedness

Coming out is conceptualized in terms of an ongoing cognitive, affective, and behavioral process. It has implications for how one thinks, feels, and behaves in relation to one's sexuality. Coming out can be examined at three levels: the intrapsychic, the interpersonal, and the intergroup.

As many models of sexual identity development postulate, LGB people come to append a label to their sexuality and then incorporate it into their sense of identity. At the intrapsychic level, therefore, coming out refers to the individual's acceptance, assimilation, and accommodation of their sexuality in their identity. This can be referred to as coming out to oneself (Markowe, 1996). Coming out can be considered an interpersonal process when the LGB person decides to share their sexual identity with another person. Indeed, the interpersonal dimension is often what people are referring to when they talk about coming out. Yet, coming out can also be thought of in terms of an intergroup process when the LGB person defines their sexuality in terms of a social identity (Tajfel & Turner, 1979), that is, a group membership and sees and presents himself or herself primarily as a member of that group and different from heterosexual people. The intergroup dimension of coming out entails telling other LGB people "I have something in common with you, share your concerns and, therefore, perceive solidarity with you" and, as some of the sexual identity development models note, telling heterosexual people "I have little or nothing in common with you, feel oppressed by you, and feel no solidarity with you." This prompts intergroup behavior, such as activism to safeguard the identity *of the group*.

Coming out—at any of these three levels—is not binary. It is rare to be completely "out" or completely "in the closet." Although LGB people are often asked whether or not they are out (in a binary manner), the answer to this question is almost always nuanced (e.g., "to some people but not to others," "my parents know but we don't talk about it much," or "I assume that people just know"). As such, one may consider oneself to be "out" to particular individuals (e.g., family members) even though they have never openly discussed their sexuality with them. Caba et al. (2022) used latent class analysis to identify different types of outness in a sample of 8884 young LGB people in the United States and found six clusters: out to all but teachers; out to siblings and peers; out to siblings and lesbian, gay, bisexual, transgender, queer, or questioning (LGBTQ) peers; out to LGBTQ peers; mostly not out; and very much not out. In an interview study of 53 gay and lesbian adults, Rossi (2010) found that interviewees typically reported coming out to a friend first and that more had come out to their mother than their father. Moreover, mothers were generally informed using direct methods while fathers were informed using indirect methods. Differences may in part be explained by the level of interest and enquiry from particular groups or individuals—Rossi (2010) found that mothers tended to enquire more about coming-out individuals' sexuality than fathers.

In contrast to the behavioral process of coming out, outness can be regarded as a state but is of course indicative of the behavioral process of coming out. It essentially tells us "how much" coming out has occurred. After all, as one comes out to more people and to a greater extent to each person, one's degree of outness increases. It is common for LGB people to describe themselves as "out to everyone," "out to some," "out to nobody," and so on. Conversely, the metaphors "being in the closet," "being closeted," and "closetedness" are antonyms of outness. They are used to refer to LGB people who have not yet disclosed their sexual identity to others. However, what is often actually meant is that they have not disclosed their sexual identity to particular significant others. For instance, Jaspal and Siraj's (2011) gay male interviewees described themselves as "closeted" but did report having a gay social network to whom they clearly had disclosed their sexual identity. Since they had not come out to their parents and were therefore careful about self-disclosure, they did not consider themselves to be out.

Measuring Outness

Various quantitative scales have been developed to measure degree of outness. Wilkerson et al. (2016) make the case for use of a single-item measure of outness: "I would say that I am open (out) as gay, bisexual, or a man attracted to other men." Although they found that the single-item measure performed better in terms of its concurrent validity than multi-item scales of outness, the scale does not allow insight into the nuances of coming out that have been highlighted above.

Conversely, the multi-item Outness Inventory (Mohr & Fassinger, 2000) examines the degree to which the individual is out (1=person definitely does not know about your sexual orientation status to 7=person definitely knows about your sexual orientation status, and it is OPENLY talked about) to particular groups and individuals (e.g., mother, father, new straight friends, members of one's religious community). The scale can be used in three ways: first, individual items can be used to examine outness to particular groups and individuals; second, there are three factors that can be calculated to measure degree of outness in the life domains of family, everyday life, and religion; and, third, the scale can be used to provide a measure of overall outness.

The Nebraska Outness Scale (Meidlinger & Hope, 2014) was developed to examine degree of outness in terms of two constructs: disclosure and concealment of sexual orientation. The scale provides measures of how much the LGB person discloses their sexual identity and how much they conceal it. The authors found that concealment was more strongly associated with mental health outcomes than disclosure.

Significant Others

Significant others are essentially people who matter to the coming-out individual. The relationship that they have with this person constitutes a role or element of identity, such as "son," "brother," "best friend," or simply "family." As an element of identity, the relationship that one has with their significant other is powerful and can shape how the coming-out individual sees himself or herself. For instance, as noted throughout this book, a positive reaction to coming out from a significant other can motivate the individual to append positive meanings to their sexuality and to come out to others while a negative reaction can have regressive effects upon sexual identity development, priming the individual to express trepidation about coming out again. This book is concerned specifically with LGB people's experiences of coming out to significant others.

Enablers and Inhibitors of Coming Out

There are many factors that can enable or inhibit coming out in LGB people. Some of the major enabling and inhibiting factors have been examined in previous research and are discussed in this section. Three broad clusters of enablers and inhibitors of coming out can be identified: demographic factors; social factors (e.g., minority stressors and social support); and psychological factors relating to identity.

Demographic Factors

Various demographic factors have been found to influence the degree of outness (White & Stephenson, 2013). Sexual identity development milestones, including coming out to others, have been found to occur in various sequences and at different points across the life course by demographic factors, such as sex, sexual orientation, ethnicity, and birth cohort (Hall et al., 2021).

Age is a key demographic factor. Vale et al. (2019) found age to be a significant predictor of outness in their study of 228 sexual minorities aged 18–80 years, with older respondents generally reporting higher outness. However, the picture is complex—in an Italian study of LGB people (Pistella et al., 2020), it was found that younger people reported an earlier coming out experience than older people. Moreover, the nature of one's coming out experience may differ by age cohort which plausibly may affect future decision-making regarding coming out. After all, if initial experiences are negative, one may refrain from coming out to others.

van Bergen et al. (2021) conducted a qualitative thematic analysis of 155 LGB people in three age cohorts (18–25, 35–42, and 52–59). They found that, while invalidating responses from parents were common across all cohorts, validating responses were more often observable in the youngest cohort. People in the oldest cohort were generally accepting of their parents being non-communicative about their sexuality. Studies of older LGB people generally highlight the role of social and contextual factors (such as the fact that same-sex attraction was previously more stigmatized, less acknowledged, and, in some cases, criminalized) in their decision-making regarding coming out (e.g., Neville et al., 2015).

Social Factors

As highlighted throughout this book, the identity of the individual is complex and multi-faceted, consisting of multiple elements and guided by multiple principles (see Chap. 3). One's other group memberships may shape both coming out decision-making and the nature of one's coming out experience. These include ethnicity, social class, occupation, and many others (Grov et al., 2006; Jaspal & Bloxsom, 2023; Marrs & Staton, 2016; Taylor, 2009).

In particular, religion and the social representations associated with one's religious group membership have commonly been found to influence cognition, affect, and behavior in relation to coming out. For instance, in a study of Christian gay and bisexual men, Wilkerson et al. (2012) found that among Evangelical Protestants (but not Mainline Protestants or Catholics), religiosity was associated with higher internalized homonegativity which in turn was associated with lower outness. In his study of British South Asian gay men, Jaspal (2012) found that, while

Muslims generally exhibited internalized homonegativity, fearing divine retribution, Hindus and Sikhs conversely expressed concerns about stigmatization from others in their ethno-cultural group. Differences by religious group can be attributed to the different social representations that operate within them.

As LGB people become aware of their same-sex attraction and develop their sexual identity, they become aware of dominant social representations of LGB people. In a heteronormative society, these representations tend to stigmatize their sexuality. Moreover, they may have first-hand experiences of stigma, prejudice, discrimination, and other minority stressors due to their sexuality (Frost & Meyer, 2023). Collectively, these social representations and experiences influence coming out decision-making. For instance, in their study of LGB college students in the United States, Garvey et al. (2018) found that institutional experiences at college and, especially, perceived attitudes toward LGB people on campus were associated with their degree of outness, with negative perceived attitudes and experiences being related to less outness (see also Dentato et al., 2014). Perceived neighborhood homonegativity has been found to be associated with decreased outness in a national sample of minority ethnic LGBTQ people in the United States (Kavanaugh et al., 2020).

Experiences within family settings also appear to be key. Parental reactions to coming out (e.g., whether they support, attempt to control, or reject their child's sexuality) have been found to affect identity development and psychological wellbeing in the coming-out individual (D'Amico et al., 2015). Moreover, Little et al. (2023) found that adaptive family functioning was associated with higher outness and that this relationship was mediated by sexuality-specific support from family members (but not by general support from family members).

The family is important in part because it can provide the LGB person with the perception that they are supported. There are of course many sources of social support. For instance, in a qualitative study (Akers et al., 2021), LGB people described finding the confidence to disclose their sexual identity to others when they initiated a same-sex relationship due to the support and empowerment that they derived from their intimate partners. Furthermore, in occupational contexts, LGB people are more likely to decide to come out when they perceive greater employer support (both in terms of policies and support for them as LGB individuals) and, in these contexts, coming out is associated with positive outcomes, such as job satisfaction and lower job anxiety (Griffith & Hebl, 2002). Jaspal (2025a, 2025b) also found general social support to be associated with increased outness in samples of LGB people in the United Kingdom.

Some LGB people derive social support using the Internet which can be perceived as a "safe space" in which they can manage the disclosure of their sexuality. The availability of the Internet can be considered a facilitator of coming out for some LGB people. In their qualitative study of LGBTQ youth, Craig and McInroy (2014) found that the new media, such as websites, web-based television and news, social media, social networking platforms, and video sharing, enabled coming-out individuals to access resources, to explore their identities, to connect with others who share their identity, to come out digitally, and to extend their coming out from online to offline settings. However, Bond et al. (2009) found that heavy users of social media were less likely to communicate openly about their sexuality with their families but that they were able to fulfill psychological needs, such as social support and self-esteem, through their social media use.

In his qualitative study, Giano (2021) highlights the benefits of online experiences for coming-out gay men, arguing that online experiences expedite the coming out process by facilitating early milestones regarding the realization of their sexuality and helping them to affirm a LGB identity, as well as facilitating engagement with other LGB people. Lovelock (2019) examined coming out narratives on YouTube and found that these videos provided an opportunity for authentic self-presentation and for the disclosure of what it feels like to be LGB in a heteronormative context, while also ensuring the visibility of LGB identities. Owens (2017) examined the Facebook profiles of young adult gay men and found that, while some used the platform to celebrate and affirm their gay identity, others used it to share their gay identity with some but not others. In short, social networking platforms may allow LGB people to manage their coming out strategically.

Identity Factors

As indicated by the sexual identity development models, LGB people who develop a strong sexual identity at both the intrapsychic and group levels appear to be more likely to come out to others. Indeed, in their study of 2401 lesbian women, Morris et al. (2001) found that three lesbian identity variables (lesbian self-identification, number of years self-identifying as a lesbian, and involvement in the LGB community) were associated with higher outness. Consistent with this argument, Whitman and Nadal (2015) found that negative identity variables in relation to being LGB (e.g., internalized homonegativity and identity confusion) were generally associated with less outness. Similarly, Jaspal (2025a, 2025b) found that positive sexual identity variables, such as sexual identity salience and sexual identity certainty, were positively associated with outness, while negative variables, such as internalized homonegativity, sexual identity threat, and anticipating homonegativity from others, were inversely associated with outness.

Empirical research shows that more general positive identity variables that are not necessarily related to one's sexuality are also associated with higher outness. This is why the total identity of the coming-out individual is so important. For instance, in their study of gay men, Jaspal and Breakwell (2022) found that identity resilience (the perception that one's identity is characterized by higher levels of self-esteem, self-efficacy, continuity, and positive distinctiveness) was indirectly associated with higher degree of outness through lower perceived stigmatization of one's sexuality. Moreover, in their study of 311 LGB people in the United States, Goshorn et al. (2022) found that aspects of self-compassion (specifically lower self-isolation, higher self-kindness, and lower self-judgment) and the search for meaning in life were associated with higher outness.

The Benefits and Pitfalls of Coming Out

A key focus of this book is on the benefits and pitfalls of coming out from the perspective of LGB people themselves. In previous research, outness has generally been found to be associated with various positive social, psychological, and even physical health outcomes (Ballester et al., 2021; Bejakovich & Flett, 2018; Jaspal & Breakwell, 2022; Lopes & Jaspal, 2024). Moreover, as shown in Chap. 2, the sexual identity development models tend to position coming out to others as the hallmark of a positive sexual identity characterized by high levels of psychological wellbeing.

The reported benefits of coming out are manifold. Perrin-Wallqvist and Lindblom (2015) used interpretative phenomenological analysis to understand experiences of adolescents' coming out. Despite initial challenges, such as feelings of alienation, uneasiness, and fear, interviewees generally reported self-acceptance, feeling comfortable with their sexuality, and feeling whole in the aftermath of coming out. The experience of coming out was largely construed as liberating.

Outness also appears to be good for physical health outcomes. In their study of 150 lesbian and bisexual women, Tabaac et al. (2015) found that outness was associated with wellness behaviors (e.g., regular exercise, engagement with primary care, and nutrition habits) through higher perceived social support and lower depression. A study of 4901 gay, bisexual, and other men who have sex with men in 13 cities in the European Union found that outness was associated with higher likelihood of human immunodeficiency virus (HIV) testing and of being reached by HIV prevention programs (Gios et al., 2021). In a study of 2401 lesbian women, higher outness was inversely associated with psychological distress and suicidality (Morris et al., 2001).

There is evidence that outness is beneficial for interpersonal relationships. Using qualitative methods, Akers et al. (2023) found that outness was associated with higher relationship satisfaction among LGB people in a same-sex relationship. Similarly, in his interview study with 20 gay couples, LaSala (2000) found that outness was perceived as beneficial for the relationship primarily because individuals did not need to conceal the relationship and could involve their partners in family events and activities.

Yet, coming out is often preceded by fear and anxiety in view of the uncertainty surrounding other people's reactions (Perrin-Wallqvist & Lindblom, 2015). Some of these fears are unfortunately realized. Johnston and Jenkins (2004) examined accounts of coming out in mid-adulthood from a sample of gay and lesbian older people. Participants' accounts showed that coming out could disrupt social relationships, induce fear of losing important things and people and, particularly, interact with religion to produce a sense of oppression. Interviewees highlighted the need for courage and strength in order to cope effectively but some also acknowledged their engagement in maladaptive, self-destructive behaviors to attempt to cope.

There is also evidence that, under particular psychological and social conditions, coming out may actually be conducive to poor mental health outcomes. For example, Riggle et al. (2017) found degree of outness to be a statistically significant predictor of increased depressive symptoms which they attributed to the increased likelihood of exposure to discrimination and other minority stressors when coming out. It should be noted that in their study higher sexual identity concealment was also associated with higher depressive symptoms, indicating the dilemmatic position occupied by LGB people in contexts that are not affirmative of their sexuality.

Furthermore, Ryan et al. (2015) surveyed 108 LGB people regarding their first coming out experiences and found that a negative reaction was associated with both higher depression and lower self-esteem. Incidentally, positive reactions did not account for additional variance in the wellbeing variables. Specifically, when the negative reactions were associated with decreased autonomy support (i.e., support to be oneself), they were in turn associated with higher depression and lower self-esteem (see also Legate et al., 2012). Moreover, Rentería et al. (2023) found that, while outness was generally associated with higher self-esteem and lower depression in their study, LGB people who were still questioning their identity (i.e., those with increased sexual identity uncertainty) reported higher depression in the aftermath of coming out. In their study of 400 young LGB adults in France, Charbonnier and Graziani (2016) found that stress characterized the coming out process for most respondents due to two factors: fear of causing distress to loved ones (by coming out) and the perception that coming-out individuals themselves had limited resources to cope.

Chang et al. (2021) provide insight into the pathways between outness and mental health outcomes. They found that outness was associated with decreased depressive symptoms through the mediation of social support, suggesting that, when outness generates access to social support, which is of course not always the case, LGB people experience less depression. In their study, outness was also associated with more severe mental health conditions (i.e., borderline personality disorder) through both social support and discrimination, suggesting that, when outness provides social support, the risk of poor mental health decreases. Conversely, when outness exposes LGB individuals to more discrimination the risk of poor mental health increases.

The pitfall of negative reactions from significant others has also been observed in experimental research. Breakwell and Jaspal (2022) conducted an experiment with 333 gay men in which half were asked to recall and describe a negative coming out experience to someone significant and half to recall and describe a positive coming out experience. Those who recounted a negative coming out experience reported higher identity threat and psychological distress than those who recounted a positive experience. Identity resilience and internalized homonegativity moderated these relationships, suggesting that identity resilience may buffer the effects of threat and that internalized homonegativity may accentuate them upon recall of a negative coming out experience.

Using the same design but with a sample of LGB people, Lopes and Jaspal (2024) found that, in both conditions, minority stressors, such as discrimination and rejection, were associated with higher identity threat and psychological distress, while protective factors, such as identity resilience and social support, were associated with less threat and distress. The valence of the coming out experience (negative vs positive) moderated these effects, with the effects of minority stressors being accentuated in the negative recall condition. Thus, it appears that, when LGB people recall a negative reaction to a previous coming out experience, everyday minority stressors (e.g., discrimination) may become more salient and have adverse effects on mental health. A negative reaction from a significant other may have cumulative negative psychological effects long after the actual coming out event itself.

Notwithstanding the challenges associated with coming out, some research shows that LGB people who experience such challenges may overcome them over time. Vaughan and Waehler (2010) describe the concept of coming out growth, which refers to the identity development that can occur following the experience of psychological stress in relation to coming out to others. The concept consists of an individual dimension, whereby coming-out individuals perceive growth in relation to their self-construal, and a collectivistic dimension that includes improvement in their relationships with others. In their study, greater outness and involvement in the LGB community were associated with greater growth.

Coming Out as a Social Representation

As LGB people contemplate coming out to others, they draw on their pre-existing perceptions of what coming out entails. This process of course evolves as individuals themselves evolve, for example, through engagement with other people. Social representations theory (Moscovici, 2000) postulates that an abstract idea (e.g., the concept of coming out) acquires an essence through the processes of anchoring (i.e., linking something new to something we already know about) and objectification (i.e., making something more "concrete" through the use of personification, metaphors, and symbols), which in turn enables people to think and talk about it. The abstract idea becomes what is referred to in the theory as a social representation. A social representation consists of many elements that converge in defining the "essence" of the concept (Lahlou & Abric, 2011). Social representations in turn inform individual attitudes that determine how that concept is evaluated.

The act of coming out and, by extension, the state of outness can be viewed as social representations. There are many sources of social representation, including the media, film, literature, social media, political speeches, legal documents, medical handbooks, academic textbooks, and, crucially, everyday conversations. The sexual identity development models generally postulate that LGB people develop more positive social representations of their sexuality by engaging with these sources of information, such as seeking literature regarding their sexuality and developing friendships with other LGB people (see Chap. 2). Earlier in this chapter, the Internet and particularly social media were described as potential facilitators of coming out.

Role models also play a key role in social representations. For instance, Forenza (2017) conducted interviews with 10 "out and proud" gay men in the United States and asked them to reflect upon the role of gay icons in popular media culture in their own sexual identity development. Participants generally expressed a sense of identification with gay icons and indicated that the affirmative, validating messages that they received from them enabled them to come out in their own lives. Moreover, Gomillion and Giuliano (2011) examined the influence of media role models on LGB identities in both cross-sectional quantitative survey and in-depth qualitative interview studies. They found that role models in the media and the pride, inspiration, and comfort derived from them shaped participants' own self-construal as LGB as well as their coming out decision-making. Thus, LGB icons can imbue the prospect of coming out with a positive value, that is, people develop a positive social representation of it. This in turn enables them to come out.

The coming out experiences of celebrities, including actors, singers, television presenters, athletes, and politicians who were previously thought to be heterosexual, have received much media attention. For instance, when British Olympic diver Tom Daley came out as bisexual in 2013, the media generally emphasized his bravery and positioned him as a role model for young LGB people (Magrath et al., 2017). In his analysis of an interview with Thomas Beattie, a British professional footballer who came out as gay in 2020, Magrath (2025) describes the transformative coming out effect, whereby coming out is said to engender positive changes in the life of the coming-out individual. Celebrities' coming out stories are represented not only as an act of bravery but, more importantly, as the "right" thing to do. They are lauded, congratulated, and represented as exemplary LGB people. Their authenticity is celebrated.

Indeed, as shown in Chap. 5, one of the most significant positive features of coming out is framed by LGB people themselves in terms of identity authenticity. Authenticity constitutes a social value. Scholars have noted the "value-ladenness of all assessments of authenticity" (Strand, 2014, p. 60). It is both a "virtue" and a "character ideal" (Guignon, 2008, p. 286). It is represented as something that individuals should strive to achieve (Vannini & Williams, 2009). Yet, this often implies that those who are not out are, at best, living inauthentically and, at worst, living a lie. Indeed, those who are closeted may be perceived as "leading a double life," "hiding their true self," and, in some cases, deceiving others (Jaspal, 2017). Arguably, the sexual identity development models themselves position LGB people who conceal their sexuality as having an "incomplete" sexual identity.

There are many ramifications of this social representation. Those who are not out may feel stigmatized as "inauthentic" and, in some cases, be overtly denigrated by others (both heterosexuals and other out LGB people) who view their lack of outness as a flaw (Jaspal, 2017). It should be noted that not everyone possesses the social and psychological resources that are often needed to come out. Some LGB people live in deeply homonegative societies. In some countries, LGB people face persecution, violence, or even death. The positive social representation of outness is thus a double-edged sword: on the one hand, it can be inspiring and empowering for the LGB person contemplating self-disclosure and, on the other hand, it constructs closetedness as a flaw in the LGB person's identity which itself can become a source of marginalization and low self-esteem.

Coming Out in Context

LGB people come out in particular social contexts. Social context, in part, shapes the expectations and outcomes of their coming out experience. Each social context is characterized by different social representations. LGB people come out in the family home, at work, at school, at university, in sports teams, in urban settings, in rural settings, and many other contexts (Annes & Redlin, 2012; Gray, 2013; Heatherington & Lavner, 2008; Marrs & Staton, 2016; White et al., 2021). They also come out in particular cultural systems. These cultural systems vary in the extent to which they accept, or even recognize, LGB identities. In some countries, for instance, homosexuality is criminalized and even punishable by death. This does not mean that LGB people never come out in these contexts but rather that the experience of doing so is different (see, e.g., Jaspal, 2014b; Jaspal et al., 2024). The two empirical studies of coming out reported in this book draw upon the accounts of LGB people based in the United Kingdom. Most self-identified as White British. The data therefore cannot represent the experiences of all LGB people who come out. They represent just one subsection of this vastly diverse global population. Some observations about the United Kingdom context are therefore necessary for understanding the findings of these studies.

Coming Out in the United Kingdom

Like many other Western industrialized countries, the United Kingdom has made significant strides in promoting equal rights for lesbian, gay, bisexual, and transgender (LGBT) people. By international standards, the United Kingdom is considered to be among the most advanced in the world in relation to LGBT rights. In 2025, the LGBT Equality Index ranked the United Kingdom 30th of 197 countries in view of its relatively high ratings on three indices (scored out of 100): equality (69/100), legislation (82/100), and public opinion (56/100) (Equaldex, 2025). A YouGov survey of 1708 adults in the United Kingdom showed that 84% of respondents would be either very or somewhat supportive of their child, sibling, or close family member if they came out as LGB (YouGov, 2021).

A detailed analysis of the history of LGBT rights in the United Kingdom is beyond the scope of this book but there are several texts that provide this (e.g., Behrens & Becker, 2023; Jaspal, 2019; Jennings, 2007; Weeks, 2016). Some key milestones can be identified. Homosexuality was decriminalized in the United Kingdom with the Sexual Offences Act which received Royal Assent in 1967. Soon after this, the Gay Liberation Front was formed in the 1970s as a pressure group to advocate for LGBT visibility, and the first Gay Pride event was held in London in July 1972. This period also saw the establishment of gay bars, clubs, and other social venues in London and other major cities in the 1970s which provided safe spaces for LGBT people. However, the growing rights of LGBT people were curtailed with Section 28 of the Local Authority Act 1988, which stated that the local authority "shall not intentionally promote homosexuality or publish material with the intention of promoting homosexuality" or "promote the teaching in any maintained school of the acceptability of homosexuality as a pretended family relationship." Section 28, promulgated in the context of the HIV/AIDS crisis that mainly affected gay and bisexual men, generally led to a silencing of LGB identities in schools, undoubtedly shaping the meanings of coming out for many LGB people (Jaspal & Bayley, 2020).

The Stonewall Lobby Group campaigned effectively for the repeal of Section 28 in 2003, the inclusion of homophobic hate crime in the Criminal Justice Act 2003, and the promulgation of the Civil Partnership Act 2004 which provided gay and lesbian couples with the equivalent of civil marriage. The Civil Partnership Act 2004 was perhaps the most significant development in LGB rights since the decriminalization of homosexuality in 1967. Nine years later, the Marriage (Same Sex Couples) Act 2013 legalized same-sex marriage in England and Wales. Moreover, in employment settings, LGB people are protected against discrimination, harassment, and victimization due to their sexual orientation under the Equality Act 2010 which recognizes sexual orientation as one of nine "protected characteristics." Amid these significant legislative developments, Gay Pride remains an annual event in most major cities in the United Kingdom. Moreover, LGBT History Month has been observed annually since 2005 and hundreds of events (e.g., exhibitions, study days, public lectures, and film screenings) take place each year to celebrate LGBT lives, identities, and rights.

It has been argued by commentators that the United Kingdom generally offers an affirmative social and legal environment in which LGB people can come out, with some now questioning the significance of coming out as LGB. This question is returned to later in this chapter.

Global Perspectives

Most research into coming out has been conducted in Western countries, such as the United Kingdom and United States. There are, however, some studies of coming out in other country contexts which highlight possible cultural differences in relation to coming out as LGB.

Studies conducted in East Asian societies generally highlight the centrality of social relationships and particularly the family in coming out. For instance, in their interview study of fifteen gay and lesbian people's coming out experiences in Islamic Malaysia, Cheah and Singaravelu (2017) identified three themes: disclosure as self-acceptance; concealment to protect the self and others; and the construal of sexual identity as a private, not a public, identity. Overall, the findings highlight the significance of relationships with other people, particularly significant others, and personal safety in decision-making regarding coming out. The primary aim appears to be the protection of valued interpersonal relationships. Similarly, in their analysis of 60 Chinese gay men's coming out stories, Bie and Tang (2016) found that the decision to come out, the way in which their gay identity was disclosed and communicated about, and the aftermath of coming out were all shaped by Chinese cultural values, such as family, marriage, and sense of duty to others. Wang et al. (2009) interviewed Taiwanese gay men regarding their coming out experiences. Their findings indicated that coming out decision-making was shaped in part by individuals' perception of their parents' attitudes toward homosexuality and that they strove to come out in ways that would minimize the negative impacts of identity disclosure, acknowledging that their parents, in some cases, had their own experience of coming out as the parents of a gay person.

There has also been some research into aspects of coming out in Middle Eastern societies, which generally shows that coming out is associated with threats to psychological wellbeing due mainly to the impact upon significant others (Jaspal et al., 2024). Maatouk and Jaspal (2023) conducted a survey of 200 gay and bisexual men in Lebanon. They found that outness was associated with higher levels of internalized sexual orientation stigma (i.e., homonegativity in gay men and binegativity in bisexual men). In another study of gay and bisexual men in Lebanon, Assi et al. (2025) found that outness was associated with higher anxiety, which they attributed to the fear associated with negative reactions to their sexuality. Jaspal (2014b) conducted an interview study with Iranian gay men who had migrated to the United Kingdom. He found that, despite the very challenging social and legal conditions for LGB people in Iran, some interviewees reported having come out to others and accepted that they would be stigmatized due to their sexuality. They had come to terms with the stigma that existed and sought opportunities for enacting their sexual identity in "safe" ways, that is, by avoiding detection by the authorities. Despite migration to the United Kingdom, some still experienced identity threat and poor mental health due to the magnitude of the minority stressors that they had experienced in Iran. Their accounts clearly demonstrated the lasting impact for identity processes.

Ethnic and Religious Minorities

Studies have also examined coming out among LGB people of ethnic and religious minority backgrounds who are living in Western societies. One focus of these studies has been on the ways in which sexuality interacts with these other elements of identity to shape the coming out experience.

In their interview study of progressive Muslim gay men in the United States, Minwalla et al. (2005) found that the perceived negative effect of coming out upon their families, including their siblings, was a key consideration. Similarly, several studies of gay men of Pakistani Muslim origin in the United Kingdom show that the perception that their religion and sexuality are fundamentally incompatible can create significant conflict in identity (referred to as threats to psychological coherence) and reduce the likelihood of coming out to family members (Jaspal, 2014a; Jaspal & Cinnirella, 2010, 2012, 2014). Siraj (2011, 2012) has found similar themes in her research into Muslim lesbian women.

This does not necessarily mean that Muslim LGB people do not come out but rather that perceived stigma, especially from family members, may lead to strategic decision-making about the management of coming out. Indeed, in their interview study of British Muslim gay men who had not yet come out, Jaspal and Siraj (2011) found that, although individuals were fearful of coming out due to the shame that they felt that it would bring on their families, they viewed coming out as a possible future strategy for coping with the threats to identity that they experienced. In other words, they aspired to come out—in a culturally appropriate way—to live out their gay identities. Incidentally, coming out has also been found to be challenging for British Indian gay men which may be attributed to cultural, rather than religious, pressures (Jaspal, 2012, 2014a).

There have also been studies of Black and Latino LGB people in the United States that show the significance of ethnicity and culture in coming out. For instance, in their longitudinal study of coming out in an ethnically diverse sample of LGB people in the United States, Rosario et al. (2004) found that Black and Latino LGB people were less likely to be out than White LGB people and postulated that cultural factors might delay the integration of a LGB identity in the self and coming out to others. Sexual identity development models would view these cultural factors as an impediment to progressing beyond the initial stages of identity development. Moreover, in their study of Black lesbian and bisexual women in the United States, Bowleg et al. (2008) found that decision-making about coming out was shaped by familial, community, and religious factors, rather than by a personal desire to be more out.

Gerena (2023a) conducted a systematic review of studies in the United States examining Latino gay men's experiences of coming out to their fathers specifically. Studies generally indicated that Latino gay men anticipated, and often encountered, a negative reaction from their fathers which could be attributed to machismo but also the centrality of family identity and family roles. Yet, a cohesive family identity could also operate as a protective factor when coming out. Negative reactions were generally associated with feelings of shame and poor mental health. In his own empirical study of Latino gay men using phenomenological approaches, Gerena (2023b) has also observed that interviewees report fear of rejection from their families and especially from their fathers, which could be attributed to pervasive cultural norms that stigmatize homosexuality. Individuals in his study reported coping maladaptively with this fear by consuming alcohol as an escapist strategy (see also Jaspal, 2021).

LGB people of ethnic minority background face stressors due not only to their sexuality (e.g., homonegativity) but, in some cases, also to their ethnicity (i.e., racism) (Jaspal, 2017). Stanton et al. (2019) found that both naturalized citizens and non-citizens of the United States who identified as LGBT were less likely than citizens to be out in private and public spheres, while controlling for other demographic factors. This suggests that a precarious citizenship status can shape coming out decision-making. Similarly, Lewis (2012) shows how migration can sometimes facilitate and impede coming out, with some LGB people feeling pressured to return to the closet following migration (cf. Jaspal, 2014b).

Another minority stressor faced by some LGB people is that of sexual racism, which is defined as "a specific form of racial prejudice enacted in the context of sex or romance" (Callander et al., 2015, p. 1991). LGB people may be rejected by potential romantic or sexual partners due to "sexual preferences" for particular races (i.e., not theirs), which can undermine self-esteem (Thai, 2020). Sexual racism also has been found to affect decision-making regarding coming out. In a study of 80 minority ethnic gay and bisexual men in the United States (Ma et al., 2025), it was found that higher exposure to sexual racism was associated with lower outness to one's family. This suggests that exposure to a distal stressor due to another minority identity (in this case, ethnicity) can shape decision-making regarding coming out as LGB.

Is Coming Out Still Relevant?

Despite the evidence presented above, some of which has been generated in Western societies, some commentators have been questioning the relevance of coming out in a so-called "post-gay" society. Savin-Williams (2005) argued that LGB youth in Western industrialized countries, such as the United Kingdom and the United States, now live in the "post-gay" era in which LGB people have gained societal acceptance to the extent where "gay adolescents have the same developmental concerns, assets, and liabilities as heterosexual adolescents" (p. 222). In view of increased societal acceptance, post-gay theorists argue that LGB people are less inclined to perceive their sexuality as a central element of their identity and thus do not feel the need to come out (Ghaziani, 2014; McCormack et al., 2015). Indeed, Savin-Williams (2005, p. 1) argues that

> teenagers are increasingly redefining, reinterpreting, and renegotiating their sexuality such that possessing a gay, lesbian, or bisexual identity is practically meaningless. Their sexuality is not something that can be easily described, categorized, or understood apart from being part of their life in general.

Savin-Williams (2005) also postulates that young LGB people are reluctant to label themselves as LGB and that their sexual identity is expressed fluidly. Some researchers have also noted the "softening" of masculinities in a post-gay era, whereby young men are increasingly comfortable with expressing same-sex affection, not only because social representations of masculinity are changing but also because of the fluidity of sexual self-identification and declining significance of homonegativity (e.g., McCormack, 2012; McCormack & Anderson, 2010). Moreover, Ghaziani (2011) argues that the post-gay era has also shaped intergroup relations and that the previous "us vs them" discourse of opposition is increasingly displaced by the discourse of inclusion, namely "us and them," with implications for LGBT activism.

The material presented in this book challenges the post-gay concept. There is evidence that the majority of young LGB people do continue to lay claim to traditional sexual identity categories (Russell et al., 2009), which is also reiterated by the accounts of coming-out LGB people presented in this book. Weststrate and McLean (2010) conducted an interesting study in which 251 gay and lesbian people were asked to relate a memory of a cultural event or a self-defining memory relating to their sexuality. Younger participants were more likely than older participants to report a self-defining memory (such as a significant coming out experience), indicating the continued significance of LGB identity for younger people. Chandra (2022) similarly notes that LGB identities remain meaningful for many same-sex attracted individuals—especially for those from ethnic minority backgrounds for whom a post-gay world may appear to be a distant utopian future (see also Jaspal & Siraj, 2011).

The broader social repercussions of the post-gay concept should also be considered. In his book *The Rise and Fall of Gay Culture*, Harris (1997, p. 4) writes that

> By looking closely at the changes that have occurred in gay culture in the past few decades, I attempt to represent the process through which a culture with unique traditions and rituals is submerged into the melting pot, its distinguishing characteristics dissolving into this grey, flavorless gruel as its members are accepted by society at large.

Harris (1997) views post-gay culture as a loss of identity and fears that, amid the "normalization" of LGB identities, their distinctiveness will be lost. As post-gay theorists argue, in many Western societies "lesbian and gay people experience greater freedom, rights, and autonomy regardless of sexuality" (Mathers et al., 2018, p. 2) and "same-sex attracted people are said to have largely achieved social, institutional, and legal equality" (Lea et al., 2015, p. 1266). These developments must of course be celebrated. However, they cannot and must not be assumed to reflect the lived experience of all LGB people, many of whom do not enjoy this level of equality and continue to experience coming out as socially and psychologically challenging.

Kampler and Connell (2018) provide an excellent critique of the post-gay concept, highlighting the dangers of this discourse. As they note, the post-gay concept "defines an entire generation via the experiences of a small number of privileged gays and lesbians (young, urban-dwelling, educated, wealthy, partnered, normatively gendered, and White) to the exclusion of the many who cannot or will not leverage their resources" to live in accordance with it (p. 7). Lewis (2023) similarly provides a compelling critique of the concept, noting that it offers a promise of utopia and disingenuously provides an illusion of inclusion obviating the need for systemic change in what are actually heteronormative and, in some cases, homonegative societies.

Using the MTV teen series *Faking It* as a case study, Monaghan (2021, p. 428) shows how the post-gay politics of "tolerance, acceptance and genuine love" can conceal a dangerous politics of normalization that itself masks the stigma, prejudice, and discrimination that many LGB people continue to face. Discourse possesses an action orientation (Edwards & Potter, 1992). Post-gay discourse promotes the erroneous belief that homonegativity is no longer a problem and that actions to challenge it are thus unnecessary. Yet, the many studies using minority stress theory clearly demonstrate the multitude of stressors faced by LGB people due to their sexual identity (see Frost & Meyer, 2023). Thus, in contrast to claims of the declining significance of homonegativity, the voices of over 500 LGB reproduced in this book people show that homonegativity persists and continues to shape the coming out experience. In some cases, homonegativity is subtle but no less insidious than its traditional forms. Coming out *is* relevant.

Overview of the Book

This book focuses upon the effects of coming out for identity processes in LGB people. Chapter 2 provides a review of seminal models of sexual identity development. In view of the limitations associated with these models, an alternative theoretical model predicting the degree of outness is proposed. Chapter 3 outlines the major tenets of identity process theory and minority stress theory from social psychology and suggests that the integration of these theories can shed light upon the psychological aspects of coming out and especially the impact that the interpersonal dimension of coming out can have for the total identity of the individual. Chapter 4 provides an overview of the methodological aspects of the two empirical studies reported in this book and highlights the need for triangulation of empirical findings to provide more comprehensive insights into the psychology of coming out.

The next five chapters describe the major themes arising from the written and interview accounts of the LGB people who participated in the two empirical studies. Chapter 5 focuses upon the association of coming out to significant others with the derivation of identity authenticity. Chapter 6 examines the positive implications of coming out for interpersonal relationships, including the continuity and strengthening of bonds between the coming-out individual and their significant others. Chapter 7 explores the negative implications of coming out for interpersonal relationships, namely rejection, emotional distance, and ambiguous loss experienced in its aftermath. Chapter 8 describes the non-acknowledgement, invalidation, and silencing of LGB people's identities by significant others following the coming out event. Chapter 9 focuses on three types of psychological violence experienced by LGB people when they come out, namely microaggressions, ghosting, and gaslighting.

The final chapter of this book describes a theoretical framework, based upon the findings and contextualized within existing theory and research, within which the antecedents, consequences, and experiences of coming out as LGB can be collectively examined. The framework should inform the ways in which LGB people are supported to develop a positive sexual identity and to come out in ways that enhance their psychological wellbeing.

References

Akers, W. P., Cashwell, C. S., & Blake, S. D. (2021). Images of resilience: Outness in same-gender romantic relationships. *Journal of LGBTQ Issues in Counseling, 15*(2), 168–194. https://doi.org/10.1080/15538605.2021.1914272

Akers, W. P., Cashwell, C. S., & Blake, S. D. (2023). Relationship satisfaction and outness: The impact of the closet on connection. *Sexual and Relationship Therapy, 38*(4), 813–833. https://doi.org/10.1080/14681994.2021.1937597

Anderson-Carpenter, K. D. (2022). Do spirituality, rurality, and LGBTQ support increase outness and quality of health in gay and bisexual men? *Journal of Homosexuality, 69*(6), 1081–1096. https://doi.org/10.1080/00918369.2021.1905382

Annes, A., & Redlin, M. (2012). Coming out and coming back: Rural gay migration and the city. *Journal of Rural Studies, 28*(1), 56–68. https://doi.org/10.1016/j.jrurstud.2011.08.005

Assi, M., Jaspal, R., Newman, K., & McDermott, D. (2025). Depression, anxiety, and life satisfaction in gay and bisexual men in Lebanon: A cross-sectional correlational study. *Sexuality and Culture*. https://doi.org/10.1007/s12119-025-10394-5

Ballester, E., Cornish, M. A., & Hanks, M. A. (2021). Predicting relationship satisfaction in LGBQ+ people using internalized stigma, outness, and concealment. *Journal of GLBT Family Studies, 17*(4), 356–370. https://doi.org/10.1080/1550428X.2021.1923104

Behrens, P., & Becker, S. (Eds.). (2023). *Justice after stonewall: LGBT life between challenge and change*. Routledge. https://doi.org/10.4324/9781003286295

Bejakovich, T., & Flett, R. (2018). "Are you sure?": Relations between sexual identity, certainty, disclosure, and psychological well-being. *Journal of Gay & Lesbian Mental Health, 22*(2), 139–161. https://doi.org/10.1080/19359705.2018.1427647

Bie, B., & Tang, L. (2016). Chinese gay men's coming out narratives: Connecting social relationship to co-cultural theory. *Journal of International and Intercultural Communication, 9*(4), 351–367. https://doi.org/10.1080/17513057.2016.1142602

Bond, B. J., Hefner, V., & Drogos, K. L. (2009). Information-seeking practices during the sexual development of lesbian, gay, and bisexual individuals: The influence and effects of coming out in a mediated environment. *Sexuality & Culture, 13*(1), 32–50. https://doi.org/10.1007/s12119-008-9041-y

Bowleg, L., Burkholder, G., Teti, M., & Craig, M. L. (2008). The complexities of outness: Psychosocial predictors of coming out to others among Black lesbian and bisexual women. *Journal of LGBT Health Research, 4*(4), 153–166. https://doi.org/10.1080/15574090903167422

Breakwell, G. M. (1986). *Coping with threatened identities*. Methuen.

Breakwell, G. M., & Jaspal, R. (2022). Coming out, distress and identity threat in gay men in the United Kingdom. *Sexuality Research & Social Policy, 19*(3), 1166–1177. https://doi.org/10.1007/s13178-021-00608-4

Caba, A. E., Mallory, A. B., Simon, K. A., Rathus, T., & Watson, R. J. (2022). Complex outness patterns among sexual minority youth: A latent class analysis. *Journal of Youth and Adolescence, 51*(4), 746–765. https://doi.org/10.1007/s10964-022-01580-x

Callander, D., Newman, C. E., & Holt, M. (2015). Is sexual racism really racism? Distinguishing attitudes toward sexual racism and generic racism among gay and bisexual men. *Archives of Sexual Behavior, 44*(7), 1991–2000. https://doi.org/10.1007/s10508-015-0487-3

Chandra, S. (2022). A multi-faceted and relational approach to gay men's identities. *Sociology, 56*(6), 1070–1086. https://doi.org/10.1177/00380385221081389

Chang, C. J., Kellerman, J. K., Fehling, K. B., Feinstein, B. A., & Selby, E. A. (2021). The roles of discrimination and social support in the associations between outness and mental health outcomes among sexual minorities. *American Journal of Orthopsychiatry, 91*(5), 607–616. https://doi.org/10.1037/ort0000562

Charbonnier, E., & Graziani, P. (2016). The stress associated with the coming out process in the young adult population. *Journal of Gay & Lesbian Mental Health, 20*(4), 319–328. https://doi.org/10.1080/19359705.2016.1182957

Cheah, W. H., & Singaravelu, H. (2017). The coming-out process of gay and lesbian individuals from Islamic Malaysia: Communication strategies and motivations. *Journal of Intercultural Communication Research, 46*(5), 401–423. https://doi.org/10.1080/17475759.2017.1362460

Craig, S. L., & McInroy, L. (2014). You can form a part of yourself online: The influence of new media on identity development and coming out for LGBTQ youth. *Journal of Gay & Lesbian Mental Health, 18*(1), 95–109. https://doi.org/10.1080/19359705.2013.777007

D'Amico, E., Julien, D., Tremblay, N., & Chartrand, E. (2015). Gay, lesbian, and bisexual youths coming out to their parents: Parental reactions and youths' outcomes. *Journal of GLBT Family Studies, 11*(5), 411–437. https://doi.org/10.1080/1550428X.2014.981627

Dentato, M. P., Craig, S. L., Messinger, L., Lloyd, M., & McInroy, L. B. (2014). Outness among LGBTQ social work students in North America: The contribution of environmental supports and perceptions of comfort. *Social Work Education, 33*(4), 485–501. https://doi.org/10.1080/02615479.2013.855193

Edwards, D., & Potter, J. (1992). *Discursive psychology*. Sage.

Equaldex. (2025). *LGBT equality index. The most LGBT-friendly countries in the world.* Accessed May 10, 2025, from https://www.equaldex.com/equality-index

Forenza, B. (2017). Exploring the affirmative role of gay icons in coming out. *Psychology of Popular Media Culture, 6*(4), 338–347. https://doi.org/10.1037/ppm0000117

Frost, D. M., & Meyer, I. H. (2023). Minority stress theory: Application, critique, and continued relevance. *Current Opinion in Psychology, 51*, 101579. https://doi.org/10.1016/j.copsyc.2023.101579

Garvey, J. C., Matsumura, J. L., Silvis, J. A., Kiemele, R., Eagan, H., & Chowdhury, P. (2018). Sexual borderlands: Exploring outness among bisexual, pansexual, and sexually fluid undergraduate students. *Journal of College Student Development, 59*(6), 666–680. https://doi.org/10.1353/csd.2018.0064

Gerena, C. E. (2023a). Latino gay men's disclosure of sexual identity to their fathers: A systematic review. *Journal of Family Studies, 29*(5), 2459–2478. https://doi.org/10.1080/13229400.2022.2109983

Gerena, C. E. (2023b). The coming out experience of Latino gay men. *Families in Society, 104*(2), 101–110. https://doi.org/10.1177/10443894211039836

Ghaziani, A. (2014). *There goes the gayborhood?* Princeton University Press.

Ghaziani, A. (2011). Post-gay collective identity construction. *Social Problems, 58*(1), 99–125. https://doi.org/10.1525/sp.2011.58.1.99

Giano, Z. (2021). The influence of online experiences: The shaping of gay male identities. *Journal of Homosexuality, 68*(5), 872–886. https://doi.org/10.1080/00918369.2019.1667159

Gios, L., Mirandola, M., Sherriff, N., Toskin, I., Blondeel, K., Dias, S., Alexiev, I., et al. (2021). Being in the closet. Correlates of outness among MSM in 13 European cities. *Journal of Homosexuality, 68*(3), 415–433. https://doi.org/10.1080/00918369.2019.1656033

Gomillion, S. C., & Giuliano, T. A. (2011). The influence of media role models on gay, lesbian, and bisexual identity. *Journal of Homosexuality, 58*(3), 330–354. https://doi.org/10.1080/00918369.2011.546729

Goshorn, J. R., Mason, W. N., & Sperandio, K. R. (2022). Does meaning-in-life or self-compassion influence LGBTQ+ identity or outness? *Journal of LGBTQ Issues in Counseling, 16*(4), 368–389. https://doi.org/10.1080/26924951.2022.2093309

Gray, E. M. (2013). Coming out as a lesbian, gay or bisexual teacher: Negotiating private and professional worlds. *Sex Education, 13*(6), 702–714. https://doi.org/10.1080/14681811.2013.807789

Griffith, K. H., & Hebl, M. R. (2002). The disclosure dilemma for gay men and lesbians: "Coming out" at work. *Journal of Applied Psychology, 87*(6), 1191–1199. https://doi.org/10.1037/0021-9010.87.6.1191

Grov, C., Bimbi, D. S., Nanín, J. E., & Parsons, J. T. (2006). Race, ethnicity, gender, and generational factors associated with the coming-out process among gay, lesbian, and bisexual individuals. *The Journal of Sex Research, 43*(2), 115–121. https://doi.org/10.1080/00224490609552306

Guignon, C. (2008). Authenticity. *Philosophy Compass, 3*(2), 277–290. https://doi.org/10.1111/j.1747-9991.2008.00131.x

Hall, W. J., Dawes, H. C., & Plocek, N. (2021). Sexual orientation identity development milestones among lesbian, gay, bisexual, and queer people: A systematic review and meta-analysis. *Frontiers in Psychology, 12*, 753954. https://doi.org/10.3389/fpsyg.2021.753954

Harris, D. (1997). *The rise and fall of gay culture*. Hyperion.
Heatherington, L., & Lavner, J. A. (2008). Coming to terms with coming out: Review and recommendations for family systems-focused research. *Journal of Family Psychology, 22*(3), 329–343. https://doi.org/10.1037/0893-3200.22.3.329
Jaspal, R. (2012). "I never faced up to being gay": Sexual, religious and ethnic identities among British South Asian gay men. *Culture, Health and Sexuality: An International Journal for Research, Intervention and Care, 14*(7), 767–780. https://doi.org/10.1080/13691058.2012.693626
Jaspal, R. (2014a). Arranged marriage, identity and psychological wellbeing among British Asian gay men. *Journal of GLBT Family Studies, 10*(5), 425–448. https://doi.org/10.1080/1550428X.2013.846105
Jaspal, R. (2014b). Sexuality, migration and identity among gay Iranian migrants to the UK. In Y. Taylor & R. Snowdon (Eds.), *Queering religion, religious queers* (pp. 44–60). Routledge. https://doi.org/10.4324/9780203753040-11
Jaspal, R. (2017). Coping with ethnic prejudice on the gay scene: British South Asian gay men. *Journal of LGBT Youth, 14*(2), 172–190. https://doi.org/10.1080/19361653.2016.1264907
Jaspal, R. (2019). *The social psychology of gay men*. Palgrave Macmillan. https://doi.org/10.1007/978-3-030-27057-5
Jaspal, R. (2021). Chemsex, identity processes and coping among gay and bisexual men. *Drugs and Alcohol Today, 21*(4), 345–355. https://doi.org/10.1108/DAT-12-2020-0083
Jaspal, R. (2025a). A theoretical model for predicting outness in lesbian, gay and bisexual people: Minority stressors, social support and identity processes. *Social Sciences, 14*(4), 207. https://doi.org/10.3390/socsci14040207
Jaspal, R. (2025b). Minority stressors, social connectedness and degree of outness in gay men: Data from two cross-sectional correlational studies in the United Kingdom. *Sexuality and Culture, 29*(3), 1318–1338. https://doi.org/10.1007/s12119-025-10325-4
Jaspal, R., & Bayley, J. (2020). *HIV and gay men: Clinical, social and psychological aspects*. Palgrave Macmillan. https://doi.org/10.1007/978-981-15-7226-5
Jaspal, R., & Bloxsom, C. (2023). Identity processes, stressors and mental health in Black, Asian and minority ethnic sexual minorities. In J. Semlyen & P. Rohleder (Eds.), *Sexual minorities and mental health: Current perspectives and new directions* (pp. 107–133). Palgrave Macmillan. https://doi.org/10.1007/978-3-031-37438-8_6

Jaspal, R., & Breakwell, G. M. (2022). Identity resilience, social support, and internalized homonegativity in gay men. *Psychology and Sexuality, 13*(5), 1270–1287. http://doi.org/10.1080/19419899.2021.2016916

Jaspal, R., & Cinnirella, M. (2010). Coping with potentially incompatible identities: Accounts of religious, ethnic and sexual identities from British Pakistani men who identify as Muslim and gay. *British Journal of Social Psychology, 49*(4), 849–870. https://doi.org/10.1348/014466609X485025

Jaspal, R., & Cinnirella, M. (2012). Identity processes, threat and interpersonal relations: Accounts from British Muslim gay men. *Journal of Homosexuality, 59*(2), 215–240. https://doi.org/10.1080/00918369.2012.638551

Jaspal, R., & Cinnirella, M. (2014). Hyper-affiliation to the religious ingroup among British Pakistani Muslim gay men. *Journal of Community and Applied Social Psychology, 24*(4), 265–277. https://doi.org/10.1002/casp.2163

Jaspal, R., Maatouk, I., & Assi, M. (2024). Identity, mental health, and coping among sexual minorities in the Middle East and North Africa: The case of Lebanon. In M. Ryan & H. Rizzo (Eds.), *Sexuality in the Middle East and North Africa: Contemporary issues and challenges* (pp. 236–258). Syracuse University Press.

Jaspal, R., & Siraj, A. (2011). Perceptions of 'coming out' among British Muslim gay men. *Psychology and Sexuality, 2*(3), 183–197. https://doi.org/10.1080/19419899.2010.526627

Jennings, R. (2007). From 'woman-loving woman' to 'queer': Historiographical perspectives on twentieth-century British lesbian history. *History Compass, 5*(6), 1901–1920. https://doi.org/10.1111/j.1478-0542.2007.00482.x

Johnston, L. B., & Jenkins, D. (2004). Coming out in mid-adulthood: Building a new identity. *Journal of Gay & Lesbian Social Services, 16*(2), 19–42. https://doi.org/10.1300/J041v16n02_02

Kampler, B., & Connell, C. (2018). The post-gay debates: Competing visions of the future of homosexualities. *Sociology Compass, 12*(12), e12646. https://doi.org/10.1111/soc4.12646

Kavanaugh, S. A., Taylor, A. B., Stuhlsatz, G. L., Neppl, T. K., & Lohman, B. J. (2020). Family and community support among sexual minorities of color: The role of sexual minority identity prominence and outness on psychological well-being. *Journal of GLBT Family Studies, 16*(1), 1–17. https://doi.org/10.1080/1550428X.2019.1593279

Kuyper, L., & Vanwesenbeeck, I. (2011). Examining sexual health differences between lesbian, gay, bisexual, and heterosexual adults: The role of sociodemographics, sexual behavior characteristics, and minority stress. *The Journal of Sex Research, 48*(2–3, 263), –274. https://doi.org/10.1080/00224491003654473

Lahlou, S., & Abric, J-C. (2011). What are the "elements" of a representation? *Papers on Social Representations*, 20, 20.1-20.10.

Lasala, M. C. (2000). Gay male couples: The importance of coming out and being out to parents. *Journal of Homosexuality, 39*(2), 47–71. https://doi.org/10.1300/J082v39n02_03

Lea, T., de Wit, J., & Reynolds, R. (2015). "Post-gay" yet? The relevance of the lesbian and gay scene to same-sex attracted young people in contemporary Australia. *Journal of Homosexuality, 62*(9), 1264–1285. https://doi.org/10.1080/00918369.2015.1037139

Legate, N., Ryan, R. M., & Weinstein, N. (2012). Is coming out always a "good thing"? Exploring the relations of autonomy support, outness, and wellness for lesbian, gay, and bisexual individuals. *Social Psychological and Personality Science, 3*(2), 145–152. https://doi.org/10.1177/1948550611411929

Lewis, N. M. (2012). Remapping disclosure: Gay men's segmented journeys of moving out and coming out. *Social & Cultural Geography, 13*(3), 211–231. https://doi.org/10.1080/14649365.2012.677469

Lewis, C. (2023). A wolf in sheep's clothing: A critical view of the post-gay in an Australian context. In D. Bridges, C. Lewis, E. Wulff, C. Litchfield, & L. Bamberry (Eds.), *Gender, feminist and queer studies: Power, privilege and inequality in a time of neoliberal conservatism* (pp. 191–202). Routledge.

Little, K. K., Lindahl, K. M., & Malik, N. M. (2023). Family functioning and youth outness: Indirect effect of sexuality specific family social support. *LGBTQ+ Family: An Interdisciplinary Journal, 19*(2), 160–174. https://doi.org/10.1080/27703371.2023.2167759

Lopes, B., & Jaspal, R. (2024). Identity processes and psychological wellbeing upon recall of a significant "coming out" experience in lesbian, gay and bisexual people. *Journal of Homosexuality, 71*(1), 207–231. https://doi.org/10.1080/00918369.2022.2111536

Lovelock, M. (2019). 'My coming out story': Lesbian, gay and bisexual youth identities on YouTube. *International Journal of Cultural Studies, 22*(1), 70–85. https://doi.org/10.1177/1367877917720237

Ma, J., Paltin, D., Miller-Perusse, M., Black, A., Baker, J. V., & Horvath, K. J. (2025). Sexual racism on geosocial networking applications and identity outness among sexual minority men in the US. *Journal of Homosexuality, 72*(2), 228–244. https://doi.org/10.1080/00918369.2024.2319621

Maatouk, I., & Jaspal, R. (2023). Internalized sexual orientation stigma and mental health in a religiously diverse sample of gay and bisexual men in Lebanon. *Journal of Homosexuality, 17*(8), 1441–1460. https://doi.org/10.1080/00918369.2022.2030617

Magrath, R. (2025). Thomas Beattie: A case study of coming out in men's professional football. *Soccer & Society, 26*(3), 395–408. https://doi.org/10.1080/14660970.2024.2444211

Magrath, R., Cleland, J., & Anderson, E. (2017). Bisexual erasure in the British print media: Representation of Tom Daley's coming out. *Journal of Bisexuality, 17*(3), 300–317. https://doi.org/10.1080/15299716.2017.1359130

Markowe, L. (1996). *Redefining the self: Coming out as lesbian*. Polity.

Marrs, S. A., & Staton, A. R. (2016). Negotiating difficult decisions: Coming out versus passing in the workplace. *Journal of LGBT Issues in Counseling, 10*(1), 40–54. https://doi.org/10.1080/15538605.2015.1138097

Mathers, L. A. B., Sumerau, J. E., & Cragun, R. T. (2018). The limits of homonormativity: Constructions of bisexual and transgender people in the post-gay era. *Sociological Perspectives, 61*(6), 934–952. https://doi.org/10.1177/0731121417753370

McCormack, M. (2012). *The declining significance of homophobia: How teenage boys are redefining masculinity and heterosexuality*. Oxford University Press.

McCormack, M., & Anderson, E. (2010). 'It's just not acceptable any more': The erosion of homophobia and the softening of masculinity at an English sixth form. *Sociology, 44*(5), 843–859. https://doi.org/10.1177/0038038510375734

McCormack, M., Wignall, L., & Anderson, E. (2015). Identities and identifications: Changes in metropolitan bisexual men's attitudes and experiences. *Journal of Bisexuality, 15*(1), 3–20. https://doi.org/10.1080/15299716.2014.984372

Meidlinger, P. C., & Hope, D. A. (2014). Differentiating disclosure and concealment in measurement of outness for sexual minorities: The Nebraska Outness Scale. *Psychology of Sexual Orientation and Gender Diversity, 1*(4), 489–497. https://doi.org/10.1037/sgd0000080

Minwalla, O., Rosser, B. R. S., Feldman, J., & Varga, C. (2005). Identity experience among progressive gay Muslims in North America: A qualitative study within Al-Fatiha. *Culture, Health & Sexuality, 7*(2), 113–128. https://doi.org/10.1080/13691050412331321294

Mohr, J., & Fassinger, R. (2000). Measuring dimensions of lesbian and gay male experience. *Measurement and Evaluation in Counseling and Development, 33*(2), 66–90.

Monaghan, W. (2021). Post-gay television: LGBTQ representation and the negotiation of 'normal' in MTV'S faking it. *Media, Culture & Society, 43*(3), 428–443. https://doi.org/10.1177/0163443720957553
Morris, J. F., Waldo, C. R., & Rothblum, E. D. (2001). A model of predictors and outcomes of outness among lesbian and bisexual women. *American Journal of Orthopsychiatry, 71*(1), 61–71. https://doi.org/10.1037/0002-9432.71.1.61
Moscovici, S. (2000). *Social representations: Explorations in social psychology*. Polity.
Neville, S., Kushner, B., & Adams, J. (2015). Coming out narratives of older gay men living in New Zealand. *Australasian Journal on Ageing, 34*(S2), 29–33. https://doi.org/10.1111/ajag.12277
Owens, Z. D. (2017). Is it Facebook official? Coming out and passing strategies of young adult gay men on social media. *Journal of Homosexuality, 64*(4), 431–449. https://doi.org/10.1080/00918369.2016.1194112
Perrin-Wallqvist, R., & Lindblom, J. (2015). Coming out as gay: A phenomenological study about adolescents disclosing their homosexuality to their parents. *Social Behavior and Personality: An International Journal, 43*(3), 467–480. https://doi.org/10.2224/sbp.2015.43.3.467
Pistella, J., Caricato, V., & Baiocco, R. (2020). Coming out to siblings and parents in an Italian sample of lesbian women and gay men. *Journal of Child and Family Studies, 29*(10), 2916–2929. https://doi.org/10.1007/s10826-019-01597-0
Rehman, Z., Lopes, B., & Jaspal, R. (2020). Predicting self-harm in an ethnically diverse sample of lesbian, gay and bisexual people in the United Kingdom. *International Journal of Social Psychiatry, 66*(4), 349–360. https://doi.org/10.1177/0020764020908889
Rentería, R., Feinstein, B. A., Dyar, C., & Watson, R. J. (2023). Does outness function the same for all sexual minority youth? Testing its associations with different aspects of well-being in a sample of youth with diverse sexual identities. *Psychology of Sexual Orientation and Gender Diversity, 10*(3), 490–497. https://doi.org/10.1037/sgd0000547
Riggle, E. D. B., Rostosky, S. S., Black, W. W., & Rosenkrantz, D. E. (2017). Outness, concealment, and authenticity: Associations with LGB individuals' psychological distress and well-being. *Psychology of Sexual Orientation and Gender Diversity, 4*(1), 54–62. https://doi.org/10.1037/sgd0000202

Rosario, M., Schrimshaw, E. W., & Hunter, J. (2004). Ethnic/racial differences in the coming-out process of lesbian, gay, and bisexual youths: A comparison of sexual identity development over time. *Cultural Diversity & Ethnic Minority Psychology, 10*(3), 215–228. https://doi.org/10.1037/1099-9809.10.3.215

Rossi, N. E. (2010). "Coming out" stories of gay and lesbian young adults. *Journal of Homosexuality, 57*(9), 1174–1191. https://doi.org/10.1080/00918369.2010.508330

Russell, S. T., Clarke, T. J., & Clary, J. (2009). Are teens "post-gay"? Contemporary adolescents' sexual identity labels. *Journal of Youth and Adolescence, 38*(7), 884–890. https://doi.org/10.1007/s10964-008-9388-2

Ryan, W. S., Legate, N., & Weinstein, N. (2015). Coming out as lesbian, gay, or bisexual: The lasting impact of initial disclosure experiences. *Self and Identity, 14*(5), 549–569. https://doi.org/10.1080/15298868.2015.1029516

Savin-Williams, R. C. (2005). The new gay teenager. *Harvard University Press.* https://doi.org/10.4159/9780674043138

Siraj, A. (2011). Isolated, invisible, and in the closet: The life story of a Scottish Muslim lesbian. *Journal of Lesbian Studies, 15*(1), 99–121. https://doi.org/10.1080/10894160.2010.490503

Siraj, A. (2012). "I don't want to taint the name of Islam": The influence of religion on the lives of Muslim lesbians. *Journal of Lesbian Studies, 16*(4), 449–467. https://doi.org/10.1080/10894160.2012.681268

Stanton, M. C., Rozas, L. W., & Asencio, M. (2019). Citizenship status matters: A social factor influencing outness among a diverse national sample of LGBT individuals. *The British Journal of Social Work, 49*(3), 722–741. https://doi.org/10.1093/bjsw/bcy079

Strand, M. (2014). Authenticity as a form of worth. *Journal for Cultural Research, 18*(1), 60–77. https://doi.org/10.1080/14797585.2013.851833

Tabaac, A. R., Perrin, P. B., & Trujillo, M. A. (2015). Multiple mediational model of outness, social support, mental health, and wellness behavior in ethnically diverse lesbian, bisexual, and queer women. *LGBT Health, 2*(3), 243–249. https://doi.org/10.1089/lgbt.2014.0110

Tajfel, H., & Turner, J. C. (1979). An integrative theory of intergroup conflict. In W. G. Austin & S. Worchel (Eds.), *The social psychology of intergroup relations* (pp. 33–48). Brooks/Cole.

Taylor, Y. (2009). Complexities and complications: Intersections of class and sexuality. *Journal of Lesbian Studies, 13*(2), 189–203. https://doi.org/10.1080/10894160802695361

Thai, M. (2020). Sexual racism is associated with lower self-esteem and life satisfaction in men who have sex with men. *Archives of Sexual Behavior, 49*(1), 347–353. https://doi.org/10.1007/s10508-019-1456-z

Vale, M. T., Pasta, P. M., & Bisconti, T. L. (2019). Exploring how age predicts outness and internalized homophobia in a lifespan sample of sexual minorities. *Innovation in Aging, 3*(Suppl 1), S304. https://doi.org/10.1093/geroni/igz038.1115

van Bergen, D. D., Wilson, B. D. M., Russell, S. T., Gordon, A. G., & Rothblum, E. D. (2021). Parental responses to coming out by lesbian, gay, bisexual, queer, pansexual, or two-spirited people across three age cohorts. *Journal of Marriage and Family, 83*(4), 1116–1133. https://doi.org/10.1111/jomf.12731

Vannini, P., & Williams, J. P. (2009). Authenticity in culture, self, and society. In P. Vannini & J. P. Williams (Eds.), *Authenticity in culture, self, and society* (pp. 1–20). Routledge.

Vaughan, M. D., & Waehler, C. A. (2010). Coming out growth: Conceptualizing and measuring stress-related growth associated with coming out to others as a sexual minority. *Journal of Adult Development, 17*(2), 94–109. https://doi.org/10.1007/s10804-009-9084-9

Wang, F. T. Y., Bih, H., & Brennan, D. J. (2009). Have they really come out: Gay men and their parents in Taiwan. *Culture, Health & Sexuality, 11*(3), 285–296. https://doi.org/10.1080/13691050802572711

Weeks, J. (2016). *Coming out: The emergence of LGBT identities in Britain from the 19th century to the present*. Quartet Books.

Weststrate, N. M., & McLean, K. C. (2010). The rise and fall of gay: A cultural-historical approach to gay identity development. *Memory, 18*(2), 225–240. https://doi.org/10.1080/09658210903153923

White, D., & Stephenson, R. (2013). Identity formation, outness, and sexual risk among gay and bisexual men. *American Journal of Men's Health, 8*(2), 98–109. https://doi.org/10.1177/1557988313489133

White, A. J., Magrath, R., & Emilio Morales, L. (2021). Gay male athletes' coming-out stories on Outsports.com. *International Review for the Sociology of Sport, 56*(7), 1017–1034. https://doi.org/10.1177/1012690220969355

Whitman, C. N., & Nadal, K. L. (2015). Sexual minority identities: Outness and well-being among lesbian, gay, and bisexual adults. *Journal of Gay & Lesbian Mental Health, 19*(4), 370–396. https://doi.org/10.1080/19359705.2015.1038974

Wilkerson, J. M., Smolenski, D. J., Brady, S. S., & Rosser, B. R. S. (2012). Religiosity, internalized homonegativity and outness in Christian men who have sex with men. *Sexual and Relationship Therapy, 27*(2), 122–132. https://doi.org/10.1080/14681994.2012.698259

Wilkerson, J. M., Noor, S. W., Galos, D. L., & Rosser, B. R. (2016). Correlates of a single-item indicator versus a multi-item scale of outness about same-sex attraction. *Archives of Sexual Behavior, 45*(5), 1269–1277. https://doi.org/10.1007/s10508-015-0605-2

YouGov (2021). *YouGov survey results.* Accessed May 12, 2025, from https://d3nkl3psvxxpe9.cloudfront.net/documents/LGBT_support_survey.pdf

2

Theoretical Approaches to Coming Out

Seminal Models of Coming Out

Over the years, many models have been proposed and a comprehensive review of them all is beyond the scope of this book. In this section, some seminal models that purport to explain aspects of the coming out process, focusing primarily on the development of sexual identity at the psychological level, are described and reviewed.

Cass' (1979) Model of Homosexual Identity Formation

Cass' (1979) model of homosexual identity formation is undoubtedly the most influential. The model postulates that, prior to constructing a homosexual identity, the individual views himself or herself as "nonhomosexual and heterosexual" because they are "socialized by and into a society that is antihomosexual and heterosexual in its outlook" (Cass, 1979, p. 222). The identity of the individual is said to be strongly influenced by the social structure of the culture in which they are socialized and thus they tend to view heterosexuality or complete sexual abstinence as the only acceptable routes for sexual self-expression. The model

R. Jaspal, *The Psychology of Coming Out*,
https://doi.org/10.1007/978-3-032-02599-9_2

outlines six subsequent stages that the individual passes through in order to construct a homosexual identity:

- In the *identity confusion* stage, the individual acknowledges that they are attracted to the same sex and that homosexuality is therefore relevant to them and/or to their behavior. At this stage, the individual expresses doubts about their heterosexuality but has not yet committed to a lesbian or gay identity. They are still questioning their sexual orientation. Yet, the recognition that they may be gay or lesbian generates cognitive and affective incongruence. They may therefore deny their homosexuality and dismiss their same-sex attraction as a phase or view their sexual orientation as something that could change. They continue to self-categorize as heterosexual. This can be attributed in part to dominant heteronormativity and, in some cases, homonegativity to which the individual is exposed either directly or indirectly. The individual is motivated to identify in ways that provide a positive sense of identity and, in view of stigmatizing social representations of homosexuality, they may be inclined to deny their sexuality and continue self-identifying as heterosexual despite their attraction to the same sex. On the other hand, some individuals in this stage begin seeking information to clarify their doubts about their sexual orientation, such as consulting books, discussing the topic of homosexuality, and engaging with therapy. In this stage, self-disclosure (i.e., coming out to others) is rare as the individual attempts unilaterally to make sense of their identity.
- In the *identity comparison* stage, the individual entertains the possibility of self-identification as gay or lesbian while examining the broader implications of self-identification in this way. Cass (1979, p. 225) states that "[t]his marks the first tentative commitment to a homosexual self." The confusion experienced in the previous stage is reduced. As they contemplate the social implications of being gay or lesbian, the individual tends to feel isolated in the identity comparison stage. They perceive an incongruence between their self-perception as gay or lesbian and others' perceptions of their sexuality. They experience alienation. They may have negative beliefs and feelings about their sexual orientation which is referred to as internalized homonegativity

(Williamson, 2000) and feel that they do not belong because of their difference (Rejiester, 2014). To address these psychological challenges, the individual may engage in passing as heterosexual (i.e., feign heterosexuality), resist the stigma directed at them by devaluing what others think, suppress their homosexuality, or compartmentalize their homosexuality to separate it from other elements of identity.

- In the *identity tolerance* stage, the individual becomes aware that there are other people who share their sexuality and they begin to seek contact with them to address the feelings of self-isolation and alienation that they experience in the identity comparison stage. Although they feel more certain of their sexual orientation, they may not be ready to adopt a gay or lesbian identity. As they engage with other gay or lesbian people, they will be exposed to more favorable social representations of their sexuality and acquire the linguistic tools to talk about a possible gay or lesbian identity. They no longer feel as alienated as in the previous stage because others who share their sexuality expose them to more positive images of it. The quality of contact with other gay and lesbian people is significant—those that are positive may undo the individual's negative perception of being gay or lesbian while those that are negative may accentuate the incongruence experienced in previous stages. In this stage, feelings of internalized homonegativity may begin to wane, enhancing the individual's self-image, but perceived differences between gay/lesbian and heterosexual people may be accentuated. This may lead to further self-distancing from heterosexual people.
- In the *identity acceptance* stage, the individual not only tolerates but actually accepts their gay or lesbian identity. It is "normalized" as an acceptable element of identity. They are no longer fearful of self-identifying as gay or lesbian and continue to engage with other gay or lesbian people. This can further accentuate perceived differences between their own sexual ingroup and heterosexual people. They continue to be exposed to favorable images of their sexual orientation. The gay and lesbian subculture now plays an important role in the individual's life and, to avoid the previously experienced incongruence associated with homonegativity, they may increase contact with other gay and lesbian people and decrease that with heterosexuals. Yet, as

they deepen their association with other gay and lesbian people, they strive to carve a space for themselves within that community.

- In the *identity pride* stage, the individual not only accepts but also positively evaluates their gay or lesbian identity. Having been exposed to favorable images of their sexual orientation, they now perceive it as an element of identity and derive feelings of pride on the basis of this identity element. In the identity pride stage, being gay or lesbian is perceived not only as an individual trait but also as a group membership. Gay and lesbian people are immersed in the gay and lesbian community and may no longer associate with heterosexual people. In some cases, they reject heterosexual people and their institutions and values. This in turn enables the lesbian or gay individual to reject the homonegativity habitually directed at them by heterosexuals whose opinions now matter less. Disclosure of one's sexual identity (or coming out at the interpersonal level) is a significant aspect of this developmental stage. This is said to create more situations in which the individual's identity can be validated and also align the individual's private and public identities. The impact of reactions to one's coming out is acknowledged in the model, with positive reactions facilitating further identity development and negative reactions possibly arresting it.
- In the *identity synthesis* stage, the individual integrates their sexuality into their overall sense of self which consists of other identity elements. One's sexuality is no longer perceived as the only identity element, although it remains important, but rather is synthesized with these other identity elements. At the intergroup level, perceived hostility from heterosexuals, encapsulated by the "us vs them" mentality, decreases and the individual accepts that their identity is accepted by at least some heterosexuals. The individual comes to perceive similarities between himself/herself and heterosexuals because their sexual identity is not the only frame of reference. It is but one element of an identity consisting of many others.

Although the model remains influential, it has faced much criticism over the years. First, the model implies that gay and lesbian people pass through all six stages in order to achieve identity synthesis. However, it is likely that not all the stages are necessarily significant for all gay and lesbian people—people may experience some but not all of them. Moreover, individuals may go through the stages in a different order, potentially returning to earlier stages. For instance, having achieved identity acceptance, an event may occur that leads the individual once again to experience confusion regarding their sexuality.

Second, as a psychological model, there is a focus upon the individual's cognition and affect in relation to their sexuality with little attention to the role of socio-cultural factors that are known to shape cognition, affect, and behavior. As noted in Chap. 1, culture plays an important role in the construction and management of sexual identity and, thus, it is reasonable to predict that a same-sex attracted person would progress through the stages differently in particular social and cultural contexts. For instance, a same-sex attracted person socialized in a deeply religious society may find it more challenging to derive identity pride on the basis of their sexuality, due to the higher risk of internalized homonegativity, than a person socialized in a secular context (see Maatouk & Jaspal, 2023).

Third, the model does not account for the role of minority stressors that operate at social/institutional (e.g., discrimination, rejection) and intrapsychic (e.g., internalized homonegativity, stigma anticipation) levels. These stressors too influence how the individual constructs their lesbian, gay, or bisexual (LGB) identity and can have different effects for a person's willingness to come out (see Jaspal, 2025a).

Finally, there is limited attention to the interpersonal process of coming out, that is, disclosure of one's sexuality to others. This is presented as an element of the identity pride stage but not elaborated upon. Indeed, this particular criticism can be levelled against at most of the sexual identity development models reviewed in this chapter.

Troiden's (1989) Model of Homosexual Identity Development

Drawing upon many of the insights presented in the Cass (1979) model, Troiden (1989) proposed a developmental model of homosexual identity formation that maps onto the individual's development from childhood to adulthood. The model consists of four stages.

- In the *sensitization* stage, which occurs before puberty, the child becomes aware of their difference from their same-sex peers which may indicate that homosexuality is personally relevant to them. Crucially, at this stage, the individual does not yet construe himself or herself as gay or lesbian. They may feel that they do not conform to particular gender expectations, such as playing football in the case of young boys or playing with dolls as in the case of young girls. The model suggests that, due to dominant social representations in Western societies, such as those of the United States and the United Kingdom, that tend to link gender-inappropriate interests and behaviors with homosexuality, the individual who does not conform to gender expectations may begin to see homosexuality as personally relevant and believe that others doubt their heterosexuality as a result of their gender non-conformity. They believe that they may not be perceived as heterosexual by their same-sex peers and, in some cases, are teased by them. As a result, they feel marginalized.
- The *identity confusion* stage generally occurs during mid-adolescence. In this stage, the individual retrospectively recognizes that the feelings that they had during the sensitization stage were indeed indicators of their sexual orientation. They reach the conclusion that they are probably gay or lesbian but this creates dissonance between previously held beliefs about the self and those emerging in the present. The individual experiences doubts about their identity, oscillating between heterosexual and gay or lesbian identities. Social stigma is said to contribute to feelings of identity confusion since the individual wishes to be accepted but realizes that being gay or lesbian may result in rejection. When faced with identity confusion, the individual uses varied strategies that operate mainly at the cognitive level since identity disclosure tends not to have taken place yet. These strategies include denial, repair, avoidance, redefinition, or acceptance. Acceptance of one's gay or lesbian identity can enable the individual to progress to the next stage.
- In the *identity assumption* stage, which generally occurs in late-adolescence and early adulthood, the individual tolerates and sometimes accepts that they are gay or lesbian. They may engage in same-sex sexual experimentation, associate with other gay and lesbian people,

and explore sexuality-specific subcultures. It is at this stage that the individual comes out to other people. Moreover, favorable contact with other gay and lesbian people makes the prospect of belonging to a gay and/or lesbian community attractive and, consequently, the individual may come to define their sexuality in terms of a social group membership. They may use a range of mainly interpersonal and intergroup strategies for coping with exposure to stigma, such as passing as heterosexual in some contexts and seeking affiliation to the gay and lesbian community.

- In the *commitment* stage, the individual accepts, and feels comfortable with, their gay or lesbian identity. The model defines commitment as "a feeling of obligation to follow a particular course of action" and, in this context, as "adopting homosexuality as a way of life" (p. 110). This involves adopting a lifestyle that is deemed to be compatible with their sexuality. The individual is thus in a position to enter into same-sex love relationships (in contrast to the previous stage in which only sexual experimentation is deemed acceptable). Same-sex relationship formation is seen in the model as "the onset of commitment" (p. 110). The main focus of this stage is on the development of a committed relationship although it is also noted that the gay or lesbian individual will also come out to heterosexual people as a marker of their identity commitment.

Much of the criticism leveled against Cass' (1979) model is also applicable to this model. First, the mechanisms underpinning progression from one stage to another are unclear. Troiden (1988, p. 105) does state that "[h]omosexual identity development is not a linear, step-by-step process, nor is developmental change a matter of either progress or regression" and acknowledges that "[p]rogress through developmental stages occurs in a back-and-forth, up-and-down fashion." Yet, it is unclear in the model how individuals might progress through the stages and, given that each stage builds upon the previous one and maps onto the individual's development from childhood to adulthood, a linear, static progression through stages is at least implied. Gay and lesbian people may of course progress through these stages in a different order, possibly sidestepping some stages, but the model does not provide any predictions other than linear progression. It is also unclear how linear progression from one stage to the other (e.g., identity confusion > identity assumption) would occur.

Second, the model does not appear to acknowledge the role of social and cultural factors that could influence, for instance, the level of identity confusion that one experiences. For instance, socialization in a religious context in which so-called gay conversion therapy is advocated could predictably lead a gay or lesbian person to experience prolonged identity confusion, thereby delaying their transition into the identity assumption stage.

Third, the model assumes that having a same-sex love relationship is indicative of identity commitment. There are many examples that contradict this position. For instance, some gay and lesbian people with high levels of internalized homonegativity and sexual identity uncertainty, which are not indicative of identity commitment, nevertheless embark upon same-sex love relationships (Thies et al., 2016). Similarly, not all gay and lesbian people who have assimilated and accommodated their sexuality in their identity and derive feelings of pride on the basis of it are in, or wish to be in, a same-sex love relationship. This begs the question as to the necessity of a same-sex love relationship in order to achieve identity commitment, that is, to construct a gay or lesbian identity. It should also be noted that not all gay and lesbian people who derive feelings of identity pride necessarily come out to others which is another indicator of identity commitment in the model.

Coleman's (1982) Model of the Developmental Stages of Coming Out

In his model of the developmental stages of coming out, Coleman (1982) identifies five stages that are said to be "descriptive of many of the patterns seen in individuals with a same-sex sexual identity" (p. 470). These patterns are not concerned with describing the etiology of same-sex interests and desires but rather on the psychological processes associated with awareness of these interests and desires.

- In the *pre-coming out* stage, the individual develops a preconscious awareness of their homosexual identity, that is, they have some notions of their homosexual identity but do not yet identify as gay or lesbian. Moreover, they tend to append negative value to it, reflecting the heteronormative society in which they are socialized. They may feel directly or indirectly rejected by society due to their sexuality and are therefore not yet inclined to disclose their sexuality to others. The individual tends to experience fear about involuntary disclosure of their sexuality and may exhibit poor mental health outcomes. The only way out of this psychologically aversive position is to acknowledge one's sexuality—beyond the preconscious awareness the individual in the pre-coming out stage possesses. Yet, the individual may conceal their sexuality not only as a self-protective measure but also because deflection strategies, such as denial, suppression, and repression, prevent them from acknowledging it.
- In the *coming out* stage, the individual is said to engage in self-admission regarding their sexuality and begins the process of disclosing their sexuality to others. Broadly speaking, the individual faces one of two possible reactions: acceptance or rejection. Acceptance can help embed their sexuality in identity and enhance feelings of self-esteem. Conversely, rejection can reinforce the negative value previously appended to sexuality in the pre-coming out stage, leading the individual to regress to that stage. According to the model, experiences of rejection may discourage the individual from coming out to others, especially when they are rejected by significant others, such as parents, family members, and close friends. It is therefore suggested that the gay or lesbian individual ought to take a strategic approach to coming out, electing to do so only to people likely to provide an affirmative response that can support their developmental journey.
- In the *exploration* stage, the gay or lesbian person explores and experiments with their newly constructed sexual identity and explores ways of meeting and interacting with other gay and lesbian people—both sexually and socially. This is referred to as an adolescent stage of development because gay and lesbian individuals are said to explore and experiment in a way similar to heterosexual adolescents and, in doing so, may be "making up for lost time" (Coleman, 1982, p. 476). In this

stage, gay and lesbian people may get locked into construing themselves primarily as sexual beings and may come to depend upon their sexual encounters for boosts of self-esteem. They may also be viewed by heterosexual people as being promiscuous and thus stigmatized further. The "hypersexuality" associated with this stage of coming out may leave gay and lesbian people feeling despondent about the development of strong same-sex romantic relationships. As a result, they may experience decreased psychological wellbeing.

- In the *first relationships* stage, the period of exploration is said to lose its intrigue and the gay or lesbian person now wishes to embark upon a romantic relationship with a same-sex partner primarily to derive intimacy. In this stage, they possess sufficiently high levels of self-esteem in order to do so. The model states that initial relationships in this stage can be disastrous due inter alia to the common perception among gay and lesbian people that the relationship will not work, the intensity and possessiveness of these relationships, and the sexual focus that relationships can take (over intimacy). While some gay and lesbian people come to acknowledge and address the aforementioned barriers to a healthy relationship, others revert to the exploration stage of coming out.
- In the *identity integration* stage, gay and lesbian people experience longer-term committed relationships that are more successful than in previous stages. They are better positioned to avoid the pitfalls of the first relationships stage, such as possessiveness, jealousy, and insecurity, and can respond to rejection and adverse relationship events with greater resilience. This can be attributed to the integration of one's sexuality in the broader identity structure.

Coleman's (1982) model of the developmental stages of coming out has a strong focus on negative aspects of the gay or lesbian person's sexual identity development process. It generally assumes that the sexual identity development process is fraught with problems with only limited attention to the positive psychological aspects that can emerge. For instance, the pre-coming out process is said to be generally characterized by internalized homonegativity, the exploration stage by hypersexuality, and the first relationships stage by maladaptive cognitions and behaviors that imperil relationship continuity. This can in part be attributed to the social and cultural context in which the model was developed since social attitudes toward homosexuality in the United States were less favorable and there were limited rights for gay and lesbian people. Nevertheless, the model does not provide much insight into the individual traits, such as resilience, and the social factors, such as the availability of support and community connectedness, that can enhance the coming out process.

In fact, the only positive psychological aspects that Coleman (1982) refers to are the interventions that therapists can deploy in order to support their gay and lesbian clients with the coming out process. These include facilitating an understanding of one's same-sex feelings, promoting self-acceptance, deconstructing negative myths and stereotypes about homosexuality, and facilitating exposure to positive images through strategic coming out. Yet, the model is fairly unique in that it does not assume that coming out is always the right course of action but that it should be managed carefully so that the gay or lesbian person can derive social support and favorable images of their sexuality. It acknowledges the transformative impact that a positive reaction, especially from a significant other, can have for the coming-out individual's sexual identity.

Like most other coming out models, the role of social context is alluded to but does not appear to be a key factor in explaining how people experience and progress through the stages. For instance, social representations of homosexuality would undoubtedly shape both the pre-coming out and coming out stages—contemplating being gay or lesbian in a context in which social representations of homosexuality are positive may lead the individuals to bypass the pre-coming out stage or at least to experience it differently from somebody coming out in a context in which homosexuality is heavily stigmatized.

The model does acknowledge the malleability of the coming out process, whereby some LGB individuals may, under some conditions, revert to previous stages and remain in those stages until certain issues are resolved. However, as with other models, there is ambiguity about what these conditions are, as well as the role of individual differences in determining occupancy of one stage, reversion to a previous stage, and progression to the next stage. For instance, Coleman (1982, p. 477) states that "[w]hen gay men and lesbians conceive of themselves as capable of loving and being loved, they are ready to enter this next stage of first relationships." However, the social and psychological factors that facilitate the capacity to conceive of oneself in this way remain unexplained in the model.

It is noteworthy that, despite its name, the model appears actually to be focused upon (barriers to) the development of healthy romantic relationships, rather than the process of disclosing one's sexual identity to other people per se. The interpersonal process of coming out to others is the focus of the coming out stage but tends to be overshadowed by the formation, development, and maintenance of romantic relationships in subsequent stages.

McCarn and Fassinger's (1996) Model of Lesbian Identity Formation

Some models have focused on specific LGB subgroups. In their model of lesbian identity formation, McCarn and Fassinger (1996) describe four "phases" of development, deliberately avoiding the term "stages of development." The model distinguishes between the formation of individual and group identities in relation to lesbianism and applies the four phases to these distinct levels of identity, which are said to be "reciprocally catalytic but not simultaneous" (p. 521). According to the model, the four phases are preceded by an undefined period of nonawareness of one's same-sex feelings and desire.

- In the *awareness* phase, the individual becomes aware of their same-sex feelings and that they are "different from the heterosexual norm and therefore from the predicted self" (p. 522) since the individual has hitherto perceived herself as heterosexual. At the intergroup level, the individual becomes aware that a community of lesbians exists and that they have been socialized "under heterosexist assumptions" (p. 524).
- In the *exploration* phase, the individual examines the questions that arise in the first phase and comes to develop feelings for and strong relationships with other women, some of which involve sexual exploration. At the intergroup level, the individual seeks knowledge about

other lesbians and therefore contemplates membership in that social group although she may not yet derive a sense of belonging in that group.

- In the *deepening/commitment* phase, the individual deepens her self-awareness as a lesbian and develops "clarity and commitment to her self-fulfillment as a sexual being" (p. 523). She realizes that this has implications for her identity and comes to define herself as a lesbian, adopting this label to append meaning to her sexuality. She becomes committed to a lesbian identity and rejects previous heterosexual assumptions about her identity. At the intergroup level, the individual adopts a lesbian group membership and becomes aware of the oppression faced by members of the ingroup due to their shared lesbian identity. She identifies with lesbian culture and rejects heterosexist society. In this phase, the individual will experience a blend of cognitions and emotions, including "excitement, pride, rage, and internal conflict" (p. 525).
- In the *internalization/synthesis* phase, the individual integrates lesbianism in the identity structure, having achieved complete self-acceptance as a lesbian. She perceives feelings of coherence between this and other elements of her identity, often because this phase is preceded by "many years of emotional and sexual self-exploration" that result in the resolution of previous conflicts (p. 523). Yet, the model acknowledges that, despite this full self-acceptance, the individual is careful about self-disclosure and may refrain from coming out in contexts deemed to be unsafe, such as the workplace, for instance. Similarly, lesbian group membership is integrated in the identity structure. The individual is aware of her own and other lesbians' social oppression and may become politicized to address this. The model states that internalization/synthesis at the group level precedes that at the individual level.

Unlike the other models reviewed in this chapter, McCarn and Fassinger's (1996) model focuses specifically on the development of lesbian identity. Although it shares many characteristics with these other models, there are some key differences.

The model refers to "phases" rather than "stages" "because of the greater flexibility implied" by the former (p. 521). The authors conceptualize the phases as continuous and circular, rather than unidirectional, noting specifically the role of novel relationships and social contexts in determining how the individual experiences these phases. Yet, a close examination of the model reveals that the "phases" may be less flexible than purported. For instance, the internalization/synthesis phase is explicitly referred to as the "final development stage" (p. 525), suggesting that it is in fact conceptualized as an end-state (and one that is desirable) with little or no possibility of reversion to a previous phase. However, research into lesbians with non-Western cultural backgrounds shows that individuals may move between the phases, seemingly having met all the criteria for the internalization/synthesis phase. Siraj's (2011, 2012) research into Muslim lesbian women suggests that, having apparently overcome the negative affect (e.g., guilt) associated with the perceived incompatibility of their sexuality and religion, they may once again experience negative affect due to exposure to homonegativity.

Another key difference of this model from others is the explicit acknowledgement of the four phases operating at both individual and group levels. According to the model, the individual acquires both self-awareness (i.e., of one's same-sex feelings) and intergroup awareness (i.e., of other lesbians as a community vis-à-vis heterosexuals). However, the model provides only limited insight into how the individual and group levels of the four phases fit together, stating only that "it is unlikely that one could reach the final phase of individual sexual identity development without beginning to address the group membership questions in the parallel branch of the model" (p. 523). In fact, it is difficult to see how any of the phases could operate at exclusively intrapsychic or group levels. It would be advantageous to articulate how the two levels of identity construction interact in shaping lesbian identity.

Weinberg et al.'s (1994) Model of Bisexual Identity Development

Based upon qualitative interview research with bisexual people, Weinberg et al. (1994) proposed a stage-based model to describe the development of bisexual identity, consisting of four stages:

- In the *initial confusion* stage, the individual has a heterosexual identity but begins to experience confusion about their heterosexuality because of emerging feelings of same-sex attraction despite continued attraction to members of the opposite sex. The individual becomes aware of their bisexual feelings but struggles to categorize them in terms of an identity label. They experience anxiety as they assume that their same-sex attractions mean that they are gay/lesbian while still feeling attracted to the opposite sex.
- In the *finding and applying the label* stage, the individual will engage in sexual encounters with both sexes and find them pleasurable. They may find sexual encounters with one sex more pleasurable than the other or equally pleasurable. As they become aware of the bisexual label, through social interactions, friendship, literature, therapy, and other information sources, they begin to see this as a label that could give meaning to the confusion aroused by their same-sex and heterosexual attraction. The individual may adopt the label through the encouragement of others. Yet, they are still exposed to stigma associated with bisexuality, which they may internalize. They may continue to experience confusion as they experience attractions that suggest they may be either heterosexual or gay/lesbian.
- In the *settling into the identity* stage, the individual assimilates and accommodates their bisexuality in the identity structure, deriving self-acceptance as bisexual, and perceives the bisexual identity label as an appropriate one. They now feel more comfortable with their bisexuality and evaluate it more favorably than in previous stages. Social support is said to be a key determinant of transition to this stage. Yet, they may still wonder whether their bisexuality is just a phase, particularly as they enter committed homosexual or heterosexual relationships. In some cases, relationship breakdown is associated with transition to either heterosexuality or homosexuality.
- In the *continued uncertainty* stage, the individual, despite having adopted the bisexual identity label, intermittently experiences doubts and uncertainty in relation to their bisexual identity. As in previous stages, there may be periods in which the individual engages in sexual behavior with one sex more than the other, which can further accentuate feelings of bisexual identity uncertainty. They periodically question

whether they are in fact bisexual. This is attributed in part to the limited availability of bisexual role models and of a bisexual community that can help reinforce bisexual identity. They may feel that they must be either heterosexual or gay/lesbian to derive acceptance in either group. Being in a monogamous relationship may also contribute to continued uncertainty about one's bisexual identity.

One of the most significant criticisms of Weinberg et al.'s (1994) model of bisexual identity development model is that it assumes that bisexual people remain in a state of continued uncertainty in relation to their sexual identity. The model implies that their identity is unstable and that this causes continual confusion. The authors attribute this perpetual state of uncertainty, albeit experienced to varying degrees across the four stages, to the lack of role models, bisexual community, and social support, which might ordinarily militate against identity doubts and uncertainty.

Yet, empirical studies suggest that perpetual identity uncertainty is not necessarily the case. For instance, Brewster and Moradi (2010) examined the personal, relational, and community aspects of bisexual identity in emerging, early, and middle adult cohorts of bisexual men and women. They found evidence of increasing identity commitment across early and middle adulthood relative to emerging adulthood, suggesting greater identity stability over time. Moreover, Kassaras and Kordouthis (2025) conducted three studies of "individuals who experience sexual and/or romantic attraction to more than one gender" (p. 98) and developed the Multisexual Identity Scale on the basis of these data. They found that many subfactors of the scale, including identity intersection/holistic growth, lesbian, gay, bisexual, and transgender (LGBT) community involvement, rejection of a monosexual identity, and understanding a multisexual identity, were associated with less sexual identity uncertainty. This suggests that, for some individuals at least, it may be the bisexual label itself (and the social representations that it evinces) that increases the risk of sexual identity uncertainty. When particular social psychological conditions are in place, individuals who experience sexual/romantic attraction to more than one sex may experience decreased uncertainty about a label that they feel adequately describes their sexuality (e.g., multisexual identity). This refutes the notion of inherent identity uncertainty implied in Weinberg et al.'s (1994) model.

A Theoretical Model Predicting Degree of Outness

All the models of sexual identity development described in this chapter offer important insights into how LGB identities are constructed. However, they are also fraught with some problems. Some of these problems can be attributed to the fact that, under close scrutiny, these models have more to say about the intrapsychic development of sexual identity and less about the interpersonal process of disclosing one's sexual identity to other people. As noted in Chap. 1, coming out can be viewed at the intrapsychic level, that is, the assimilation and accommodation of a LGB identity (coming out to oneself) and the interpersonal level, that is, the disclosure of this identity to other people (coming out to others).

Perhaps there is no straightforward way of theorizing the interpersonal process of coming out to others. After all, LGB people come out to some people but not to others, and they vary in the extent to which they come out, sharing more information with some than with others. There appear to be many factors that shape decision-making regarding coming out, some of which are not captured in existing models of sexual identity development. It is perhaps more appropriate to examine the two levels of coming out separately. After all, some people may fully assimilate and accommodate a LGB identity but choose to disclose this identity to some people or nobody at all due, for instance, to societal constraints on coming out. Others may disclose their LGB identity but continue to express doubts about it, oscillating between the many identity labels that are culturally available to them. The sexual identity development models specify a series of stages or phases that culminate in the formation of a LGB identity but tend not to theorize the relationship between the intrapsychic and interpersonal dimensions of coming out. The models generally leave two important questions unanswered, namely:

- What happens at the psychological level that in turns leads some people to come out and others to avoid doing so?
- What psychological changes are provoked as a result of coming out to others and facing a particular reaction from them?

Jaspal (2025a, 2025b) attempted to address these questions in a theoretical model to predict degree of outness in LGB people (see Fig. 2.1). In developing the model, Jaspal (2025b) first examined associations between minority stressors, aspects of social connectedness with others, and degree of outness in two cross-sectional survey studies of gay men in the United Kingdom. In the first study, the proximal stressor of internalized homonegativity was statistically significantly and negatively associated with degree of outness, when accounting for the effects of relationship status and attachment style. In the second study, the proximal stressors of internalized homonegativity and perceiving negative social attitudes toward homosexuality were negatively associated with degree of outness, while aspects of social connectedness (i.e., being in a romantic relationship and general social support) and the distal stressor of discrimination were positively associated with degree of outness.

The results appeared to reflect two key points. First, social support motivates, or perhaps empowers, gay men to come out more, which is consistent with most of the sexual identity development models reviewed above. Second, different types of minority stressors relating to their

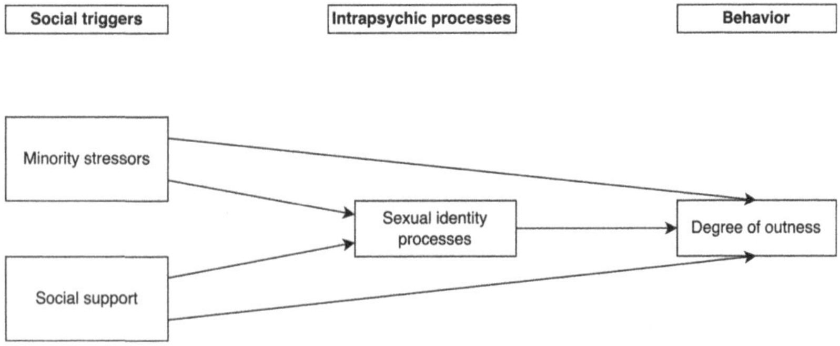

Fig. 2.1 A theoretical model for predicting degree of outness in lesbian, gay, and bisexual people

sexuality may be provoking different coming out behaviors, with distal stressors (e.g., discrimination) apparently being associated with a greater proclivity to come and proximal stressors (e.g., internalized homonegativity, the belief that most other people hold negative attitudes toward gay men), conversely, stopping gay men from doing so. This is in contrast to the sexual identity development models which tend to suggest that stigma and negative reactions to one's sexuality per se lead to decreased coming out.

It is possible that, when faced with discrimination due to their sexual orientation, LGB people may attempt to cope with this adverse social experience by seeking out identity validation and affirmation from others. To do so, they must come out—at least to some people—and probably do so strategically (Orne, 2011). It is likely that LGB people use their prior knowledge and perhaps even intuition when deciding to whom they should come out and to what extent. For instance, a LGB individual may perceive it to be safe to come out to their siblings or mother but perhaps not to their father. Furthermore, they may decide that their father need only be told that they are LGB once without any further discussion of the matter but that it is appropriate and acceptable to discuss more intimate details of their sexuality with a heterosexual friend. Strategic coming out may provide the LGB person with exposure to more favorable images of their sexual orientation from supportive others or protect them from negative images to which they might be exposed if, say, their father did not know their sexual orientation. Clearly, exposure to favorable images of one's sexual orientation may act as a buffer against the aversive experience of discrimination.

Conversely, exposure to proximal stressors, such as internalized homonegativity and perceiving negative social attitudes toward one's sexuality, appears to have more insidious effects that inhibit coming out. When a LGB person directs negative social attitudes of their sexuality toward himself or herself, they are essentially dissatisfied with this element of their identity. In fact, this may even impede the assimilation and accommodation of their sexuality in their identity and lead to perpetual "identity confusion." A person with internalized homonegativity may seek to change their sexual orientation or at least wish that they could. It is often a source of shame rather than pride (cf. Cass, 1979). Under these psychological circumstances, the LGB individual is unlikely to disclose this identity to other people.

Furthermore, the proximal stressor of perceiving negative social attitudes toward one's sexuality reflects the individual's belief that *most people* harbor negative attitudes toward this element of their identity. This is analogous to other proximal stressors that have been discussed in research using minority stress theory, such as hypervigilance (Riggle et al., 2023), stigma sensitivity (Jaspal, 2025a), and stigma anticipation (Thomeer et al., 2018). They all refer to what the individual believes others think and the expectations that they have about how they will behave toward them. This is quite different from first-hand exposure to discrimination. For instance, a LGB individual may work in a context in which homonegativity is rife and therefore face frequent experiences of discrimination due to their sexual orientation but nevertheless believe that at least some people in other contexts are accepting of their sexual identity. As such, they believe that strategic coming out could work as a strategy for counteracting the negative psychological effects of discrimination. Conversely, the belief that most people have negative attitudes toward their sexuality may lead LGB people to believe that coming out is simply unsafe. Under these psychological circumstances, remaining in the closet may therefore constitute a self-protective strategy.

Based upon the aforementioned multiple regression analyses of data from gay men, Jaspal (2025a) proposed a theoretical model of outness which he tested using structural equation modelling in two cross-sectional survey studies of LGB people in the United Kingdom. The model views the coming out process as fluid and ongoing. It occurs repeatedly across the life course as one enters novel social contexts. Identity itself (of which one's sexuality is one element) is therefore subject to revision as one engages with the social world. According to the model, there are social factors that shape the LGB person's coming-out decision-making, namely minority stressors (e.g., discrimination, rejection) and availability of social support (e.g., general social support, LGB-specific social support). The model proposes that exposure to these social factors, that is, experiencing minority stressors or believing that one is supported, provokes changes in the LGB person's identity that in turn shapes their coming-out decision-making.

In the first of two cross-sectional survey studies, Jaspal (2025a) found that perceived general social support was directly associated with greater outness and indirectly associated with outness through the mediation of higher sexual identity salience and lower sexual identity uncertainty. In other words, perceived social support was associated with a more salient sexual identity and with less uncertainty about one's sexual identity, both of which were in turn associated with greater outness. In the second study, perceived general social support was again directly associated with greater outness and indirectly though the mediation of lower sexual identity threat and lower sexual identity stigma sensitivity. Moreover, LGB-specific social support (i.e., perceived support from other LGB people) was indirectly associated with outness in similar ways to perceived general social support. However, there was no statistically significant direct relationship between LGB-specific social support and outness when the other factors were accounted for. This adds further clarification of the type of social support that LGB people may benefit from most in order to come out to others. When LGB people feel generally supported, including by heterosexual people, they may feel more empowered to come out. After all, what worries many LGB people as they contemplate coming out is a negative reaction from heterosexual people.

Across the two studies, the minority stressor of discrimination was directly associated with higher outness, supporting the hypothesis that being discriminated spurs the quest for exposure to positive images of one's sexuality through strategic coming out. However, there were also mediation effects. In the first study, discrimination was associated with higher sexual identity salience, which in turn was associated with higher outness. In the second study, discrimination was associated with higher sexual identity threat which in turn was associated with less outness. Various observations can be made about the psychological mechanisms underpinning the relationship between discrimination and outness. It was reasoned that, when an individual is discriminated against due to a particular identity element (in this case, their sexuality), this identity element appears to become more psychologically salient. In other words, it stands out more because others are drawing attention to it, albeit negatively. Incidentally, this has also been observed in studies of discrimination due to other identity elements, such as ethnicity (Hughes & Hurtado,

2018; Hurtado et al., 2015; Thompson, 1999). Identity salience in turn may make the quest for exposure to positive images in relation to this identity element all the more important, spurring greater outness (but to the right people and in the right ways). Conversely, when discrimination results in threats to sexual identity (because the discriminated LGB person now perceives decreased self-esteem, self-efficacy, continuity, and positive distinctiveness in relation to their sexuality), LGB people appear to come out less.

The studies, and the model that they test, collectively indicate that there are social factors that appear to trigger changes in sexual identity that in turn shape the LGB person's decision-making regarding coming out. Exposure to these social triggers and the experience of sexual identity change can occur at any point during the life course. This proposition is quite different from the sexual identity development models reviewed earlier in this chapter. Those models generally propose a linear developmental stage-based explanation of coming out, whereby the individual first "achieves" various positive milestones at the psychological level (e.g., identity assumption, identity pride, deepening/commitment) that in turn shape the LGB person's willingness to disclose their identity to others. As linear models, they at least imply that progression through the sexual identity development stages is unidirectional. Although the authors generally acknowledge that not every LGB individual will follow every stage or ascend through all of them in the same way, the models do not provide insight into why some stages may be followed, omitted, or prolonged. As shown in the following chapters of this book, LGB people's accounts exhibit more complexity and fluidity in these processes of sexual identity development and of coming out to other people. Furthermore, the accounts presented in this book provide more nuanced insight into the minority stressors and types of support that they may perceive upon coming out to people that matter.

The theoretical model to predict degree of outness sheds some light on the psychological changes that can occur when one faces either a negative or a positive reaction upon coming out. A negative reaction amounts to a minority stressor (e.g., discrimination, victimization, rejection) and a positive reaction could be considered an expression of interpersonal support (e.g., acceptance, identity validation). Indeed, in their experimental study examining the effects of recalled coming out experiences in gay men, Breakwell and Jaspal (2022) found that participants who recalled a negative experience experienced higher identity threat than those who reported a positive one. Thus, the negative or positive reaction itself appears to provoke sexual identity changes, shaping the LGB individual's subsequent decision-making about coming out. In the chapters that follow, the impact of coming out to others for identity processes is examined.

Overview

This chapter provides an overview of seminal models of sexual identity development in LGB people. Some of the strengths and limitations of these models are considered. The most significant criticism of virtually all the models is the linear, stage-based approach that is either assumed or explicitly stated. The relationships between the stages remain unclear. The role of social, cultural, and institutional factors is underexplored. Crucially, it has been shown that the interpersonal process of coming out to others is insufficiently addressed in the models. An alternative theoretical model predicting degree of outness is proposed. The model postulates that social factors, such as minority stressors and social support (in their many guises), may trigger changes in identity that in turn determine the extent to which LGB people come out. The model views coming out as a fluid, ongoing process that never ceases. Sexual identity is thus subject to change as one encounters novel contexts of coming out and exposure to social factors.

References

Breakwell, G. M., & Jaspal, R. (2022). Coming out, distress, and identity threat in gay men in the United Kingdom. *Sexuality Research & Social Policy, 19*(3), 1166–1177. https://doi.org/10.1007/s13178-021-00608-4

Brewster, M. E., & Moradi, B. (2010). Personal, relational and community aspects of bisexual identity in emerging, early and middle adult cohorts. *Journal of Bisexuality, 10*(4), 404–428. https://doi.org/10.1080/15299716.2010.521056

Cass, V. C. (1979). Homosexual identity formation: A theoretical model. *Journal of Homosexuality, 4*(3), 219–235. https://doi.org/10.1300/J082v04n03_01

Coleman, E. (1982). Developmental stages of the coming out process. *Journal of Homosexuality, 7*(2–3), 31–43. https://doi.org/10.1300/J082v07n02_06

Hughes, B. E., & Hurtado, S. (2018). Thinking about sexual orientation: College experiences that predict identity salience. *Journal of College Student Development, 59*(3), 309–326. https://doi.org/10.1353/csd.2018.0029

Hurtado, S., Alvarado, A. R., & Guillermo-Wann, C. (2015). Thinking about race: The salience of racial identity at two- and four-year colleges and the climate for diversity. *The Journal of Higher Education, 86*(1), 127–155. https://doi.org/10.1080/00221546.2015.11777359

Jaspal, R. (2025a). A theoretical model for predicting outness in lesbian, gay and bisexual people: Minority stressors, social support, and identity processes. *Social Sciences, 14*(4), 207. https://doi.org/10.3390/socsci14040207

Jaspal, R. (2025b). Minority stressors, social connectedness and degree of outness in gay men: Data from two cross-sectional correlational studies in the United Kingdom. *Sexuality and Culture, 29*(3), 1318–1338. https://doi.org/10.1007/s12119-025-10325-4

Kassaras, I., & Kordoutis, P. (2025). Measuring aspects of multisexuality: Initial development of the multisexual identity scale. *Journal of Bisexuality, 25*(1), 98–141. https://doi.org/10.1080/15299716.2024.2374346

Maatouk, I., & Jaspal, R. (2023). Internalized sexual orientation stigma and mental health in a religiously diverse sample of gay and bisexual men in Lebanon. *Journal of Homosexuality, 17*(8), 1441–1460. https://doi.org/10.1080/00918369.2022.2030617

McCarn, S. R., & Fassinger, R. E. (1996). Revisioning sexual minority identity formation: A new model of lesbian identity and its implications. *The Counseling Psychologist, 24*(3), 508–534. https://doi.org/10.1177/0011000096243011

Orne, J. (2011). 'You will always have to "out" yourself': Reconsidering coming out through strategic outness. *Sexualities, 14*(6), 681–703. https://doi.org/10.1177/1363460711420462

Rejiester, N. (2014). *Perception of alienation from parents and peers during the coming out process for lesbian, gay, and bisexual individuals and self-reported attachment classifications: A preliminary investigation of the relationship between the attachment system and rejection due to sexual orientation*. PhD dissertation, Washington DC, The George Washington University, US. https://scholarspace.library.gwu.edu/concern/gw_etds/6395w731z

Riggle, E. D. B., Folberg, A. M., Richardson, M. T., & Rostosky, S. S. (2023). A measure of hypervigilance in LGBTQ-identified individuals. *Stigma and Health, 8*(4), 476–486. https://doi.org/10.1037/sah0000306

Siraj, A. (2011). Isolated, invisible, and in the closet: The life story of a Scottish Muslim lesbian. *Journal of Lesbian Studies, 15*(1), 99–121. https://doi.org/10.1080/10894160.2010.490503

Siraj, A. (2012). "I don't want to taint the name of Islam": The influence of religion on the lives of Muslim lesbians. *Journal of Lesbian Studies, 16*(4), 449–467. https://doi.org/10.1080/10894160.2012.681268

Thies, K. E., Starks, T. J., Denmark, F. L., & Rosenthal, L. (2016). Internalized homonegativity and relationship quality in same-sex romantic couples: A test of mental health mechanisms and gender as a moderator. *Psychology of Sexual Orientation and Gender Diversity, 3*(3), 325–335. https://doi.org/10.1037/sgd0000183

Thomeer, M. B., LeBlanc, A. J., Frost, D. M., & Bowen, K. (2018). Anticipatory minority stressors among same-sex couples: A relationship timeline approach. *Social Psychology Quarterly, 81*(2), 126–148. https://doi.org/10.1177/0190272518769603

Thompson, V. L. S. (1999). Variables affecting racial-identity salience among African Americans. *The Journal of Social Psychology, 139*(6), 748–761. https://doi.org/10.1080/00224549909598254

Troiden, R. R. (1989). The formation of homosexual identities. *Journal of Homosexuality, 17*(1–2), 43–73. https://doi.org/10.1300/J082v17n01_02

Weinberg, M. S., Williams, C. J., & Pryor, D. W. (1994). *Dual attraction: Understanding bisexuality*. Oxford University Press.

Williamson, I. R. (2000). Internalized homophobia and health issues affecting lesbians and gay men. *Health Education Research, 15*(1), 97–107. https://doi.org/10.1093/her/15.1.97

3

Identity: Construction, Development, and Defense

What Is Identity?

Identity can be defined as the constellation of elements (e.g., group memberships, personality traits, personal preferences, attitudes, and others) that the individual believes describe himself or herself and that, taken together as a whole, make that individual unique and distinctive from others. Identity is primarily a psychological construct. It lies in the eye of the beholder, although its content is in part influenced by society. Indeed, society makes available particular categories that may become identity elements. For instance, in some Middle Eastern societies, same-sex attracted individuals may not have access to social categories, such as lesbian, gay, or bisexual, and thus not use them to describe themselves (Jaspal et al., 2024; Murray & Roscoe, 1997; Yon-Leau & Muñoz-Laboy, 2010). Furthermore, in constructing a sense of identity, people often expect acknowledgement, recognition, and validation of their identity (Jaspal & Cinnirella, 2012a). This is of course one motivation for coming out to other people. The individual first assimilates and accommodates their sexuality (i.e., being lesbian, gay, or bisexual [LGB]) in the identity structure and then shares this information with other people, often with

R. Jaspal, *The Psychology of Coming Out*,
https://doi.org/10.1007/978-3-032-02599-9_3

the expectation and hope that their sexuality will be acknowledged, recognized, and validated. Unfortunately, one's LGB identity is not always met with approval from others, as shown throughout this book.

Identity consists of many different elements. A person may see their sexuality (e.g., being LGB) as a characteristic of their identity but also describe himself or herself as Christian, shy, a keen swimmer, a socialist, and so on. In short, one belongs to many different social groups and has many different elements that collectively define one's identity. The individual will inevitably share some of these elements with other people but it is the configuration of these elements that makes them unique and distinctive. Strictly speaking, sexuality constitutes an element of identity but in this book the term "sexual identity" is used.

Identity elements vary in their significance over time and some may disappear from the identity structure altogether while new ones become part of it. For instance, during one's college years, being a student may be the most important element of one's identity, shaping the friendships one has, the activities one engages in, and being the first (or only) thing one mentions when introducing oneself, but when one leaves college and starts working, this may cease to be an element of identity. In some social contexts, particular identity elements become salient, that is, they become more important to the individual, while others are attenuated. Some may need to be attenuated to make room for others. For instance, in a study of LGB people, it was found that being exposed to discrimination due to one's sexuality was associated with higher sexual identity salience (Jaspal, 2025a). In other words, events that occur in context, such as discrimination, can make people more aware of particular identity elements. The hierarchical structure of identity is therefore constantly in flux as one encounters novel social contexts and situations.

How Is Identity Constructed?

Identity process theory (IPT) (Breakwell, 1986, 2014, 2021, 2023; Jaspal & Breakwell, 2014) provides an integrative social psychological framework for understanding how people construct, develop, and protect their sense of identity in the face of change—both societal and individual.

According to IPT, the individual seeks to construct, maintain, and protect an identity that is unique. The theory focuses specifically upon how the individual reacts to what is referred to as a threat to identity. Throughout this book, elements of IPT are drawn upon in order to shed light on the psychological aspects of LGB people's coming out experiences and particularly on the implications of coming out for identity.

Identity Processes

A stimulus refers to an event or phenomenon that evokes a change in identity. Thinking of oneself as LGB, the prospect or actual experience of sharing this information with others (i.e., coming out), and reactions from others upon coming out can all be considered stimuli which bring about some form of change in identity. IPT postulates that, in response to exposure to stimuli that are relevant to identity (such as coming out and its associated events and experiences), the individual engages in the identity processes of assimilation-accommodation and evaluation.

Assimilation-accommodation refers to the process of absorbing novel information into the identity structure. For instance, a woman who acknowledges her same-sex attraction may come to label and perceive herself as a lesbian (assimilation). Yet, for this label to become a stable fixture within the identity structure, other modifications may need to be made (accommodation). She may need to rethink the nature of her relationship with other people, such as her family, or the significance that she appends to her religious group membership. As seen in the previous chapter, assimilation has been a key focus of most sexual identity development models but there has been limited attention to accommodation, that is, what happens to the total identity of the individual when one's sexuality has been assimilated.

Evaluation refers to the meaning and value that is appended to potential and actual elements of identity. For instance, when deciding whether to label himself as gay, a same-sex attracted man will consider the broader social representations of gay men that operate within his social context. Is this acceptable? Will I be stigmatized? What are the stereotypes that are associated with gay men? These social representations will inform, but not necessarily determine, the meaning and value that he appends to being gay (see Moscovici, 1963). Some LGB people are socialized in cultural contexts in which their sexuality is relatively acceptable but they themselves may have internalized homonegativity (i.e., a negative attitude toward their own sexual orientation). On the other hand, some LGB people are socialized in cultural contexts in which their sexuality is not only stigmatized but also criminalized but themselves hold a relatively positive attitude toward it. Mainstream models of sexual identity development postulate that, during the course of sexual identity development, the individual comes to append positive value to their sexuality but empirical research shows that, despite laying claim to a LGB identity, some LGB people do not necessarily evaluate it positively (e.g., Jaspal & Cinnirella, 2010; Siraj, 2011; Williamson, 2000). This is essentially internalized homonegativity/binegativity.

IPT posits that the individual is proactive in attempting to optimize identity processes. In other words, they endeavor to engage in assimilation-accommodation and evaluation in ways that produce favorable levels of the identity principles, namely self-esteem, self-efficacy, continuity, and positive distinctiveness. IPT focuses on the total identity of the individual and, thus, in spite of the negative value that some append to their sexuality, they may nevertheless possess an overall sense of identity (consisting of other elements) that provides appropriate levels of these identity principles.

Identity Principles

The identity principles are essentially the desirable end-states for identity. IPT refers to the following four principles of identity:

- Self-esteem reflects the individual's sense of worth and value and thus amounts to the overall attitude that the individual has of himself or herself.
- Self-efficacy is the individual's sense of competence and control.

- Continuity refers to the psychological thread that unifies past, present, and future, enabling the individual to feel that they are and will remain essentially the same person despite past and future changes in their life.
- Distinctiveness reflects the individual's belief that they are unique and positively differentiated from other people.

In studies of LGB people, other principles have been proposed. In her study of the development of lesbian identity, Markowe (1996, 2002) outlined the significance of authenticity (i.e., feeling true to oneself) and affiliation (i.e., deriving a sense of belonging, acceptance, and inclusion in relevant social groups). In a series of studies examining the assimilation-accommodation of gay identity among gay men of religious faith, Jaspal and Cinnirella (2010, 2012b, 2014) proposed the concept of psychological coherence which refers to the individual's subjective perception of compatibility between identity elements that are inter-connected. While self-esteem, self-efficacy, continuity, and distinctiveness have been found to be universally significant across many empirical studies (Breakwell, 2014), it is possible that other principles, such as psychological coherence, authenticity, and affiliation, become significant in particular social contexts. For instance, in contexts in which two identity elements become inter-connected, that is, relevant to one another, the psychological coherence principle may become important. Similarly, in contexts in which one feels the need to conceal elements of one's identity, such as being a lesbian where this identity is stigmatized, the drive for authenticity and to belong in relevant social groups may become important.

Higher levels of the identity principles are generally associated with increased psychological wellbeing (Jaspal, 2024a). Therefore, the principles of identity can also be viewed as motives—they guide the operation of identity processes. In other words, people will attempt to engage in assimilation-accommodation and evaluation in ways that protect and preferably boost the principled operation of identity processes. For instance, some same-sex attracted individuals recognize that being gay/lesbian is stigmatized and come to evaluate it negatively themselves, which amounts to internalized homonegativity (Williamson, 2000). Internalized homonegativity itself is associated with lower levels of self-esteem, self-efficacy, continuity, and positive distinctiveness (Jaspal et al.,

2023). Therefore, some eschew the assimilation-accommodation of their sexuality, perhaps viewing it as a phase or behavior, rather than as an identity. Others may assimilate their sexuality in their identity but relegate this to an inferior position in the identity structure, perceiving it as an insignificant aspect of who they are. Indeed, these strategies are reflected in some of the mainstream sexual identity development models reviewed in the previous chapter.

Identity Resilience

Recent developments in IPT have focused upon the concept of identity resilience (Breakwell, 2021; Breakwell & Jaspal, 2022; Gifford et al., 2025; Jaspal, 2025b). Identity resilience is a trait-like characteristic that refers to the individual's perception of the extent to which their identity is characterized by feelings of self-esteem, self-efficacy, continuity, and positive distinctiveness. An individual is said to have high identity resilience when they perceive overall levels of the four principles to be high. While the individual four components of identity resilience fluctuate over time and context, the overall level of identity resilience is said to remain relatively stable in the face of change. Breakwell (2021, p. 580) describes identity resilience as "the capacity of the identity to resist its invalidation, devaluation or fragmentation" in the face of hazards and identifies three key functions of it.

First, identity resilience refers to the extent to which the individual's identity can absorb changes that retain its subjective meaning, value, and integrity for that individual. In other words, a person with high identity resilience will experience less identity threat when exposed to a hazard to identity. There is growing evidence to support this assertion. In their study of recalling significant coming out experiences among gay men, Breakwell and Jaspal (2022) found that identity resilience moderated that impact of recalling a negative coming out experience on reported levels of identity threat. People with higher identity resilience reported less identity threat upon recall. This effect was replicated in a sample of LGB people (Lopes & Jaspal, 2024). It is important to note that possessing an identity with high resilience does not mean that the individual never experiences identity threat. Rather, higher identity resilience appears to be associated with less threat upon exposure to a hazard.

Second, identity resilience reflects the extent to which the individual's identity facilitates adaptive coping when faced with identity threat or uncertainty. Several studies indicate that people with higher identity resilience tend to deploy coping strategies that are more adaptive, effective, and sustainable. In their study of heterosexual and LGB Lebanese university students, Jaspal et al. (2022) found that identity resilience was positively associated with the social engagement and rethinking/planning coping styles, which are considered more adaptive than some of the deflection strategies often employed in response to threat (e.g., denial). Moreover, identity resilience has been found to predict engagement in self-protective coping behaviors that minimize the risk of exposure to hazards, such as COVID-19 and HIV and their negative sequelae for identity (Breakwell et al., 2023; Gifford et al., 2025).

Third, identity resilience refers to the extent to which the individual perceives himself or herself as capable of coping with identity threat or uncertainty, that is, their perceived ability to deploy coping strategies when needed without bringing about long-term damage to the identity structure. After all, in order for coping strategies to be used effectively in the face of threat or uncertainty, the individual must have confidence in his or her ability to use them. In their study of Indian lesbian, gay, bisexual, and transgender (LGBT) people, Parwani and Talukdar (2024) found that the relationship between minority stressors and poor mental health was mediated by coping self-efficacy, indicating that lower coping self-efficacy may lead to depleted coping ability and thus poor mental health outcomes.

Although social support has been found to be among the most effective coping strategies available to people, not all LGB people actively seek social support in relation to their sexuality, especially during earlier stages of sexual identity development, as indicated by the models reviewed in Chap. 2. They may be fearful that they will face stigma, rejection, or even abuse if they do. Identity resilience has been found to be a positive predictor of social support in sexual minorities (e.g., Jaspal & Breakwell, 2022), suggesting that having an identity that is resilient is associated with feeling more confident in one's ability to seek and secure social support. In short, the perception that one is capable of coping may itself provide greater scope for creativity in coping, thereby protecting identity from threat. An individual with higher identity resilience may believe that they have more coping strategies available to them and, thus, use the strategy (or combination of strategies) deemed to be most appropriate when faced with a potential or actual threat to identity.

Identity Doubt and Identity Threat

Events and experiences associated with coming out, such as particular reactions from significant others or even contemplating coming out to them, can lead the individual to experience changes to their identity. In some cases, the individual becomes unsure about their sense of self-esteem, self-efficacy, continuity, or positive distinctiveness—this is referred to as identity doubt. In others, they actually perceive less self-esteem, self-efficacy, continuity, or positive distinctiveness, which is referred to as identity threat.

When an individual comes out as LGB to a significant other, they will have hopes and expectations regarding that person's reaction. It is easy to see how particular types of reaction may lead to identity doubt in the coming-out individual. If the reaction stigmatizes their sexuality, this can lead the coming-out individual to doubt their self-esteem. If the reaction questions the veracity of their sexuality, they may come to question their sense of continuity. If the reaction is characterized by stereotypes regarding LGB people, their feelings of positive distinctiveness may be called into question. If the reaction frames the coming-out individual's sexuality as something that must change, they may doubt their self-efficacy as they question whether this is possible.

LGB people who come out and face a challenging reaction may face doubts about one or more identity principles depending upon many different factors, such as the nature of the reaction itself, their own identity resilience prior to experiencing the reaction, and the content of their identity. For instance, a LGB person of Muslim background who is told by their parents that they are contravening their religion and are therefore not a "true" Muslim may plausibly come to doubt their self-esteem due to the negative value appended to their sexuality ("am I a failure?") as well as their sense of continuity in relation to their exclusion from their religious group ("am I no longer a Muslim?"). Identity doubt reflects uncertainty, which itself has been found to be harmful for psychological wellbeing (Bejakovich & Flett, 2018), especially among people with higher uncertainty intolerance which is a personality trait (Lopes & Jaspal, 2025). Yet, because identity is in doubt but not yet threatened, there is likely to be greater scope for reducing the uncertainty about identity and restoring appropriate levels of the identity principles. The individual may acquire greater certainty about the identity principles by engaging with other people who affirm their sexual identity, for instance.

Identity threat is said to occur when any one of the principles (self-esteem, self-efficacy, continuity, or distinctiveness) is actually undermined by events and experiences, resulting in the subjective perception of decreased levels of these principles. Identity threat has been found to be associated with recall of a negative coming out experience (Breakwell & Jaspal, 2022; Lopes & Jaspal, 2024) and with exposure to minority stressors, such as discrimination and internalized homonegativity (Jaspal, 2025a; Jaspal et al., 2023). Identity threat is harmful for psychological wellbeing. It is positively correlated with depression, anxiety, and psychological distress, and negatively correlated with life satisfaction (Assi et al., 2025; Breakwell & Jaspal, 2022; Jaspal et al., 2023). A key distinction between identity doubt and identity threat is that the latter is characterized by certainty that one's self-esteem, self-efficacy, continuity, and/or positive distinctiveness have decreased as a result of the event or experience. When threatened, the individual does not doubt but actually believes that they have decreased self-worth; that their past, present, and future are disjointed; that they have little or no control or competence; and/or that they are no longer positively distinctive from other people.

Of course, an event or experience, such as coming out to somebody significant, may challenge just one of these principles, several of them, or all of them. A modification to identity necessitated by one principle may actually introduce full-blown threats to others. For instance, continuity may motivate the individual to come out, which would enable their own self-construal to be consistent with their self-presentation to others. (The related notion of identity authenticity is discussed in Chap. 5.) However, by doing so, the coming-out individual may also be exposed to diatribes from unsympathetic family members who believe that their sexuality is unacceptable, which could be damaging for their self-esteem.

It is important to note that an event or experience that is objectively threatening (i.e., that one might expect to undermine the principles of self-esteem, self-efficacy, continuity, and positive distinctiveness) may not be subjectively perceived as such by the individual himself or herself. Any hazard will be viewed through the lens of one's identity resilience which may militate against the threat that it could cause. For example, a LGB person with higher identity resilience may be able to resist denigrating remarks about their sexuality and therefore experience little or no challenge to their self-esteem. An individual with multiple group memberships (and thus multiple sources of social support) may not perceive their continuity to be undermined when contemplating coming out to their family because they know that they will continue to receive support from other group memberships they have.

Identity Hazards

As noted earlier in this chapter, stimuli engender changes in identity. Some stimuli can be thought of in terms of a hazard to identity. A hazard has the potential to disrupt the principled operation of identity processes. In other words, it can undermine a person's levels of self-esteem, self-efficacy, continuity, and positive distinctiveness. A person exposed to a hazard can therefore be said to occupy a threatening position (Breakwell, 1986) although they may not necessarily experience identity threat. LGB people face a multitude of hazards to identity. Despite its many benefits, coming out (and its associated events and experiences) can also be considered a hazard to identity.

Minority stress theory (Frost & Meyer, 2023; Meyer 2003) provides an integrative theoretical framework for understanding the factors associated with one's stigmatized minority identity that can bring about psychological stress and thus mental health inequalities. The theory is useful for understanding the impact of hazards, which are referred to in the theory as stressors, for identity. Minority stress theory posits that LGB people face two types of stressor:

- Distal stressors are those that originate from other people and institutions and include inter alia anti-LGB policies, discrimination, prejudice, victimization, rejection, and microaggressions due to one's sexuality.
- Proximal stressors are those that are manifested at the intrapsychic level although they are the result of the individual's socialization in a context or society that is not affirmative of their sexuality. These include stressors, such as internalized homonegativity/binegativity, stigma anticipation, hypervigilance, and sexual identity concealment.

Minority stress theory posits that exposure to these stressors causes the LGB person to experience excessive psychological stress which in turn puts their health at risk. The concept of identity hazards is used since not all of them necessarily cause psychological stress. They do, however, have the capacity to bring about identity doubt or threat. Both minority stress theory and identity process theory point to coping strategies that are said to alleviate the negative psychological effects of exposure to hazards. Frost and Meyer (2023) note that minority stress theory has been extended to examine the "psychological mediation processes that explain how stigma 'gets under the skin'" (p. 2). One significant mediating factor is that of identity threat.

It is easy to see how exposure to identity hazards could disrupt the principled operation of identity processes, leading the LGB person to derive suboptimal levels of self-esteem, self-efficacy, continuity, and positive distinctiveness. Indeed, in their study of LGB people, Lopes and Jaspal (2024) showed that the relationships between rejection and psychological distress and between stigma sensitivity and psychological distress were mediated by identity threat. In other words, exposure to these hazards was associated with higher identity threat, which in turn was associated with higher psychological distress. Similarly, Jaspal (2025a) found that discrimination was associated with higher identity threat in his study of LGB people.

The alignment of minority stress theory and identity process theory may provide more nuanced insight into the consequences of exposure to hazards, such as discrimination, rejection, internalized homonegativity, and so on. It appears that, when a hazard causes identity threat, it will lead to more negative mental health outcomes. Yet, as indicated above, not all hazards will actually be experienced as a threat by everyone. After all, people react to hazards differently. Some LGB people may be able to deploy strategies for preventing threat emanating from others by discrediting the source of discrimination or rejection, for instance. It is, however, difficult to see how hazards operating at the intrapsychic level (i.e., proximal stressors in minority stress theory) could be anything but threatening for identity. Furthermore, as noted in this chapter, identity process theory identifies a broad range of coping strategies operating at the intrapsychic, interpersonal, and intergroup levels which can be deployed when exposed to a hazard. These are discussed next.

Reactions to Threat

When faced with an actual or potential threat to identity, the individual will react by engaging in varied strategies to cope. A coping strategy can broadly be defined as any cognitive, affective, or behavioral deed whose goal is to prevent, or alleviate the effects of, a threat to identity. For instance, the LGB person who anticipates or experiences a threat to continuity due to a negative reaction from somebody important to them may preemptively or subsequently rethink what that negative response actually signifies. Does the person really think I am flawed as a person because I am LGB or are they just shocked and therefore reacting emotionally? Do they now dislike me or are they just transiently angry? Will our relationship change definitively or is this just an impulsive short-lived reaction?

The way the individual perceives the reaction and the meanings that they append to it will in turn shape the effects it has on their sense of identity. Incidentally, an individual may anticipate the threat to identity to be so great that they may decide against coming out, instead preferring to conceal their sexual identity, rather than expose themselves to identity threat. Non-disclosure of one's sexual identity may itself constitute a coping strategy.

Of course, the examples above are just two of the many possible reactions to a potential or actual threat to identity. Coping strategies are varied. According to IPT, they operate primarily at three levels: intrapsychic, interpersonal, and intergroup.

Intrapsychic Coping Strategies

Intrapsychic coping strategies are those that "operate at the level of cognitions and emotions" with important implications for action (Breakwell, 1986, p. 80). They can broadly be categorized in terms of those strategies that deflect or accept the threat or its implications.

Deflection strategies include denial of the threat or its implications (e.g., being in denial about one's sexuality) and reconstrual (e.g., reconceptualizing one's sexuality as a phase, rather than as an aspect of identity). Denial is a common means of averting threats to identity. After all, the individual only experiences threat insofar as the threat is consciously perceived. The individual's denial of their sexuality essentially protects them from threats associated with acknowledgement of it. Yet, denial of one's sexuality has been found to be associated with negative affect and this relationship is mediated by anticipated rejection from others (Thöni et al., 2024). Though effective in providing short-term respite from identity threat, denial is generally unsustainable in the long term.

Reconstrual of the potentially threatening event or situation can be advantageous in some cases. By reconstruing the meaning of a negative reaction from a significant other ("they do not really think less of me of a person; they are just surprised"), the individual may experience less identity threat. This strategy may also provide time and scope, both psychologically and interpersonally, for some form of reconciliation with their significant other. Thus, as a temporary strategy, reconstrual can be effective. Yet, reconstrual can also become a means of refusing to perceive a hazard that objectively exists and morph into denial. For instance, in their study of British Muslim gay men, Jaspal and Cinnirella (2010) found that some individuals did not deny that they were attracted to other men but reconstrued their homosexuality in terms of a (mutable) behavior rather than as an identity, which allowed them to resist stigmatized social categories, such as "gay" and "bisexual." Thus, reconstrual operated as a strategy for preventing the assimilation-accommodation of sexuality in the identity structure.

Acceptance strategies include compartmentalization of the threatening stimulus in identity (e.g., accepting that one is gay but only thinking about and enacting this identity element in gay affirmative contexts and attenuating it in other contexts); anticipatory restructuring (e.g., anticipating a negative reaction to coming out from significant others and preemptively reconsidering the significance of those people in one's identity); and compromise or fundamental changes to identity (e.g., a coming-out person may transiently or permanently attenuate the significance of their religion when coming out if this is deemed to be incompatible with, or denigrating of, their sexuality).

In his qualitative study of 17 gay male college students in the United States, Tillapaugh (2013) found evidence of compartmentalization. His participants described enacting their gay identity in contexts in which it was perceived to be safe and socially permissible to do so, such as in gay-affirmative contexts, and as adopting norms associated with heterosexuality in their interactions with their male heterosexual friends. The compartmentalization strategy involves acceptance of the stigmatized element of identity but also its recognition and management. One restricts the identity element to particular social contexts and avoids its disclosure in others. This strategy is commonly observed in relation to coming out, with some LGB people choosing to do so strategically (Orne, 2011).

When faced with uncertainty or a potential threat, the individual may begin to make anticipatory changes to their identity. In their study of British Muslim gay men about their perceptions of coming out, Jaspal and Siraj (2011) found some evidence of anticipatory restructuring of identity. Some interviewees anticipated a negative reaction from significant others and preemptively attempted to gain exposure to more positives images of their sexuality by associating with other LGB people in gay-affirmative contexts, such as bars and nightclubs. While they had previously feared the prospect of coming out and, to an extent, still did have concerns about it, some now believed that coming out was possible and that it would be manageable. As one interviewee noted, "it's possible. I mean, you can like be gay and survive really" (Jaspal & Siraj, 2011, p. 191). By identifying with a new group on the basis of their sexuality (i.e., other LGB people), individuals were able to put into place an infrastructure for buffering the adverse effects of a negative reaction to coming out. They had anticipated the threat and tried to minimize its effects for identity.

Compromise and fundamental changes to identity can reduce or extinguish threats to identity. When coming out, some LGB people are faced with the suggestion, and sometimes the forceful assertion, from others that their sexuality is a phase and they are not really LGB. In order to assuage the threat to identity represented by such invalidation of an identity element that, in many cases, they have assimilated and accommodated and are therefore sharing with significant others, they may transiently comply with this suggestion. At the psychological level, they remain aware of their LGB identity but at least in their self-presentation appear to accept the notion that their sexuality is a phase. Compromise change of this kind can limit threats to identity because the coming-out individual may not be exposed to as much stigma, potentially protecting self-esteem. Moreover, they may be able to salvage their relationship with the person to whom they are coming out, potentially protecting continuity.

Fundamental change to identity can be challenging but tends to have favorable long-term outcomes. It is an acceptance strategy in every sense of the term. LGB people of religious faith may face threats to identity that emanate from their religious group membership. They may be told that their sexuality is a sin, that they will be punished by God, that they are not authentic members of the religious group, and that through prayer they can become heterosexual. Such discourse has been observed in many different religious groups (see Jaspal, 2024b; Jaspal & Cinnirella, 2010; Lomash et al., 2018). Using a case study approach, Wood and Conley (2014) describe how religious and spiritual abuse and struggle can lead to loss of religious and spiritual identity among LBG people. In other words, religion is removed from the identity structure in order to accommodate sexuality. Some coming-out LGB people of religious faith may reconstrue the meaning of their religion and view it in spiritual terms in order to accommodate their sexuality (Jaspal & Cinnirella, 2010). By focusing upon their personal relationship with God and attenuating their relationship with institutionalized religion, the individual may thus be able to assimilate and accommodate their sexuality while evading the stigma associated with institutionalized religion. Yet, any kind of change to identity can itself be challenging. Given that one's religion may be tied to other elements of identity, such as one's family or ethnicity, the successful assimilation-accommodation of one's sexuality may come at a cost, engendering additional, unanticipated threats to identity.

Interpersonal Coping Strategies

Interpersonal coping strategies are those that involve modifications to relationships with other people. Examples include isolation, negativism, passing, and compliance.

When faced with a potential or actual threat to identity, the individual may isolate himself or herself from others. Isolation, by definition, removes the risk of being denigrated by other people and thus self-esteem can be protected. Moreover, a LGB person who views their sexuality as a threat may retain their sense of continuity through self-isolation by limiting the risk of others drawing attention to it. Johnson and Amella (2014) note that LGB people may engage in self-isolation or social withdrawal in order to cope with feelings of negative distinctiveness, their non-conformity to heterosexist norms, and their fear of rejection from others. Though the strategy may be effective in protecting the individual from threats emanating from others, it may itself introduce additional threats to identity. Self-isolation necessarily entails the reduction of social contact and thus social support. Furthermore, self-isolation would likely inhibit exposure to more positive images of one's sexuality and, thus, LGB individuals who already exhibit internalized homonegativity may experience threats to self-esteem with little recourse to other interpersonal and intergroup strategies.

Conversely, negativism refers to active conflict with others who challenge the individual's identity structure. For instance, the coming-out individual may question the integrity of a close friend who reacts negatively to their identity disclosure, transforming the threat to their own identity into an attack against the source of the threat. More generally, the credibility of people who express homonegativity toward the coming-out individual may be actively challenged and they may themselves be denigrated as homophobes. LGB people of religious faith may question dominant social representations of their sexuality that are promoted by their religious group by "queering" religious scripture (Taylor & Snowdon, 2014). This entails challenging dominant interpretations of religious scripture that stigmatize one's sexuality and establishing new criteria for evaluating one's sexuality. Clearly, this strategy involves an element of interpersonal conflict as other people's social representations (in this case, those of religious authority figures) are actively challenged. All this enables the coming-out individual to reject the criteria for a positive identity that are imposed upon them by others, thereby protecting identity from threat.

One of the most common interpersonal coping strategies used by LGB people who anticipate or actually face identity threat due to their sexuality is that of passing. This involves feigning membership of a group to which one does not really belong. Many LGB people report concealing their sexuality, especially during earlier stages of sexual identity development, and, as a consequence, actively or passively feign heterosexuality. Passing can provide some respite from identity threat associated with homonegativity because the passing LGB individual is perceived by others to be heterosexual. Though they may still be exposed to general homonegativity (e.g., disparaging remarks about LGB people), in most cases, homonegativity will not be directed at them personally. For instance, in their focus group study of LGB people, Fuller et al. (2009) found that the passing strategy enabled individuals to maintain or achieve social privilege in a heteronormative society but that they were also emotional costs, such as feelings of guilt, regret, and distress due to the decreased identity authenticity associated with the strategy.

Compliance involves acceptance of the behavioral prescriptions and expectations associated with a particular position. While this is unlikely to shield identity from threat completely, it may at least reduce the amount of threat experienced because the individual is at least living up to others' expectations. For instance, a LGB person may uncritically accept the social norms (and stereotypes) associated with their identity and behave in ways that they believe to be congruent. This can facilitate feelings of acceptance and inclusion from within the LGB community, enhancing belonging, and can also provide a sense of identity authenticity. However, the strategy of compliance may still expose the individual to homonegative remarks and observations from heterosexual people.

Intergroup Coping Strategies

Intergroup strategies refer to the creation, modification, and use of social group memberships in order to protect identity from anticipated or actual threats to identity. This can involve the management of one's group memberships, the use of social group support, and social group action.

People of course have many different social group memberships. When LGB people come out, they may begin to identify with other LGB people and develop a social identity based on their sexuality. They will still have other social group memberships, which can include a religious affiliation, their family, their neighborhood, a political group, and so on. Indeed, an identity configuration that is more complex, consisting of multiple elements (especially group memberships), may offer greater scope for creativity in coping (Breakwell, 2021). The right combination of group memberships can sometimes provide respite from identity threat.

Research into identity threat among British Muslim gay men has shown that threats to identity associated with the perceived incompatibilities between being Muslim and gay (i.e., religion vs sexuality) can sometimes be assuaged through the mobilization of national identity (i.e., Britishness) (Jaspal & Ferozali, 2021). More specifically, British Muslim gay men may resist the religious norms concerning sexuality and morality more generally by self-identifying strategically as British. This strategy in turn enables them to reject both norms and stigma that can pose threats to identity.

Furthermore, when stigmatized by their family due to their sexuality, some coming-out individuals come to disidentify with their family and instead rely upon their "chosen family" (e.g., friends, other LGB people) for social support (Nardi, 1999; Weston, 1991). This amounts to the replacement of one group membership (i.e., one's biological family) with another (i.e., one's chosen family) in order to derive the same psychological needs. It has also been noted that one's chosen family can also complement one's biological family to optimize wellbeing (Hull & Ortyl, 2019). This strategy is primarily associated with the assimilation-accommodation process of identity and involves rethinking the content of identity (i.e., social group memberships) and, in some cases, reconfiguring it in order to accommodate one's sexuality.

The principal aim tends to be the derivation of social support through one's group memberships. Lopes and Jaspal (2024) have shown perceived access to social support to be inversely associated with identity threat, suggesting that having social support to hand prevents and alleviates identity threat when faced with a hazard. As LGB people contemplate coming out to significant others and in the aftermath of coming out, they may seek varied forms of support (e.g., material, emotional support) from others. This can enable them to access positive and affirmative images of their sexuality that can replace stigmatizing images associated with heteronormative contexts. Moreover, the act of exchanging confidences with a like-minded other can enable coming-out individuals to reassess the meanings of coming out—they may feel reassured about the future after confiding in a supportive other. Indeed, it has been found that LGB community connectedness is associated with decreased feelings of sexual identity threat (Jaspal, 2025a).

Engagement with peer support groups is common and effective in enhancing self-acceptance and wellbeing among people facing threat, including among LGB people. The sexual identity development models reviewed in the previous chapter position LGB peer support as a key determinant of progression through the developmental stages. Relatedly, some people who face threat recognize that the social conditions need to change in order to prevent or assuage identity threat, both for them individually and for the social group as a whole. They may engage in social group action by joining or forming a pressure group to promote social change. In many cases, the rights now available to stigmatized minority groups have resulted from social group action. The formation of Stonewall in the United Kingdom in 1989 by activists campaigning against Section 28 of the Local Government Act 1988 is a case in point (Weeks, 2016).

Overview

This chapter outlines the major tenets of identity process theory and minority stress theory and proposes that an integration of these theoretical frameworks can shed greater light on how LGB people construct, develop, and defend their identities in the context of coming out. While the sexual identity development models outlined in the previous chapter focus upon sexual identity specifically, identity process theory can enable us to understand what happens to the total identity of the individual as they contemplate or engage in coming out and are exposed to hazards to identity. Minority stress theory provides insight into the nature of hazards to identity associated with one's sexual identity. Identity process theory identifies a series of coping strategies that LGB people may use when exposed to identity hazards associated with coming out. Coping strategies vary in their level of effectiveness in the short and long term. Some are initially risky and challenging but effective in the long term, and others are easier to implement and effective in the short term but unsustainable in the long term. Some coping strategies may be designed to prevent or alleviate a threat to identity but create new threats of their own. In this book, tenets of identity process theory and minority stress theory are applied to LGB people's accounts of coming out to significant others.

References

Assi, M., Jaspal, R., Newman, K., & McDermott, D. (2025). Depression, anxiety, and life satisfaction in gay and bisexual men in Lebanon: A cross-sectional correlational study. *Sexuality and Culture*. https://doi.org/10.1007/s12119-025-10394-5

Bejakovich, T., & Flett, R. (2018). "Are you sure?": Relations between sexual identity, certainty, disclosure, and psychological well-being. *Journal of Gay &*

Lesbian Mental Health, 22(2), 139–161. https://doi.org/10.1080/19359705.2018.1427647

Breakwell, G. M. (1986). *Coping with threatened identities.* Methuen.

Breakwell, G. M. (2014). Identity process theory: Clarifications and elaborations. In R. Jaspal & G. M. Breakwell (Eds.), *Identity process theory: Identity, social action and social change* (pp. 20–37). Cambridge University Press.

Breakwell, G. M. (2021). Identity resilience: Its origins in identity processes and its role in coping with threat. *Contemporary Social Science, 16*(5), 573–588. https://doi.org/10.1080/21582041.2021.1999488

Breakwell, G. M. (2023). *Identity: Unique and shared.* Sage.

Breakwell, G. M., & Jaspal, R. (2022). Coming out, distress and identity threat in gay men in the United Kingdom. *Sexuality Research & Social Policy, 19*(3), 1166–1177. https://doi.org/10.1007/s13178-021-00608-4

Breakwell, G. M., Jaspal, R., & Wright, D. (2023). Identity resilience, science mistrust, COVID-19 risk and fear predictors of vaccine positivity and vaccination likelihood: A survey of UK and Portuguese samples. *Journal of Health Psychology, 28*(8), 747–759. https://doi.org/10.1177/13591053231161891

Frost, D. M., & Meyer, I. H. (2023). Minority stress theory: Application, critique, and continued relevance. *Current Opinion in Psychology, 51*, 101579. https://doi.org/10.1016/j.copsyc.2023.101579

Fuller, C. B., Chang, D. F., & Rubin, L. R. (2009). Sliding under the radar: Passing and power among sexual minorities. *Journal of LGBT Issues in Counseling, 3*(2), 128–151. https://doi.org/10.1080/15538600903005334

Gifford, A. J., Jaspal, R., Jones, B. A., & McDermott, D. T. (2025). Predicting PrEP acceptability and self-efficacy among men who have sex with men in the United Kingdom: The roles of identity resilience, science mistrust and stigma. *HIV Medicine, 26*(5), 677–687. https://doi.org/10.1111/hiv.13768

Hull, K. E., & Ortyl, T. A. (2019). Conventional and cutting-edge: Definitions of family in LGBT communities. *Sexuality Research & Social Policy, 16*(1), 31–43. https://doi.org/10.1007/s13178-018-0324-2

Jaspal, R. (2024a). Identity resilience, relationships, and life satisfaction: Data from two cross-sectional survey studies in the United Kingdom. *International Journal for the Advancement of Counselling, 46*(4), 856–883. https://doi.org/10.1007/s10447-024-09578-9

Jaspal, R. (2024b). Muslim LGBTQ people. In A. E. Goldberg (Ed.), *The SAGE encyclopedia of LGBTQ studies* (2nd ed.). Sage. https://doi.org/10.4135/9781071891414.n316

Jaspal, R. (2025a). A theoretical model for predicting outness in lesbian, gay and bisexual people: Minority stressors, social support and identity processes. *Social Sciences, 14*(4), 207. https://doi.org/10.3390/socsci14040207

Jaspal, R. (2025b). Identity resilience, attachment style and life satisfaction in heterosexual and gay men: The mediating effect of body image concerns *International Journal of Social Psychology.*

Jaspal, R., Assi, M., & Maatouk, I. (2022). Coping styles in heterosexual and non-heterosexual students in Lebanon: A cross-sectional study. *International Journal of Social Psychology, 37*(1), 33–66. https://doi.org/10.1080/02134748.2021.1993117

Jaspal, R. & Breakwell, G. M. (Eds.) (2014). *Identity process theory: Identity, social action and social change.* Cambridge University Press. https://doi.org/10.1017/CBO9781139136983

Jaspal, R., & Breakwell, G. M. (2022). Identity resilience, social support and internalised homonegativity in gay men. *Psychology & Sexuality, 13*(5), 1270–1287. https://doi.org/10.1080/19419899.2021.2016916

Jaspal, R., & Cinnirella, M. (2010). Coping with potentially incompatible identities: Accounts of religious, ethnic and sexual identities from British Pakistani men who identify as Muslim and gay. *British Journal of Social Psychology, 49*(4), 849–870. https://doi.org/10.1348/014466609X485025

Jaspal, R., & Cinnirella, M. (2012a). The construction of ethnic identity: Insights from identity process theory. *Ethnicities, 12*(5), 503–530. https://doi.org/10.1177/1468796811432689

Jaspal, R., & Cinnirella, M. (2012b). Identity processes, threat and interpersonal relations: Accounts from British Muslim gay men. *Journal of Homosexuality, 59*(2), 215–240. https://doi.org/10.1080/00918369.2012.638551

Jaspal, R., & Cinnirella, M. (2014). Hyper-affiliation to the religious ingroup among British Pakistani Muslim gay men. *Journal of Community and Applied Social Psychology, 24*(4), 265–277. https://doi.org/10.1002/casp.2163

Jaspal, R., & Ferozali, R. (2021). Social representations of Britishness among British South Asian gay men. *South Asian Diaspora, 13*(2), 111–128. https://doi.org/10.1080/19438192.2020.1809767

Jaspal, R., Lopes, B., & Breakwell, G. M. (2023). Minority stressors, protective factors and mental health outcomes in lesbian, gay and bisexual people in the UK. *Current Psychology, 42*(28), 24918–24934. https://doi.org/10.1007/s12144-022-03631-9

Jaspal, R., Maatouk, I., & Assi, M. (2024). Identity, mental health, and coping among sexual minorities in the Middle East and North Africa: The case of Lebanon. In M. Ryan & H. Rizzo (Eds.), *Sexuality in the Middle East and North Africa: Contemporary issues and challenges* (pp. 236–258). Syracuse University Press.

Jaspal, R., & Siraj, A. (2011). Perceptions of 'coming out' among British Muslim gay men. *Psychology and Sexuality, 2*(3), 183–197. https://doi.org/10.1080/19419899.2010.526627

Johnson, M. J., & Amella, E. J. (2014). Isolation of lesbian, gay, bisexual and transgender youth: A dimensional concept analysis. *Journal of Advanced Nursing, 70*(3), 523–532. https://doi.org/10.1111/jan.12212

Lomash, E. F., Brown, T. D., & Paz Galupo, M. (2018). "A whole bunch of love the sinner hate the sin": LGBTQ microaggressions experienced in religious and spiritual context. *Journal of Homosexuality, 66*(10), 1495–1511. https://doi.org/10.1080/00918369.2018.1542204

Lopes, B., & Jaspal, R. (2024). Identity processes and psychological wellbeing upon recall of a significant 'coming out' experience in lesbian, gay and bisexual people. *Journal of Homosexuality, 71*(1), 207–231. https://doi.org/10.1080/00918369.2022.2111536

Lopes, B., & Jaspal, R. (2025). Exposure to ghosting, gaslighting and coercion and mental health outcomes. *Partner Abuse*. https://doi.org/10.1891/PA-2024-0031

Markowe, L. (1996). *Redefining the self: Coming out as a lesbian*. Polity.

Markowe, L. (2002). Young lesbians: Coming out into the future. *Lesbian & Gay Psychology Review, 3*(1), 11–18. https://doi.org/10.53841/bpslg.2002.3.1.11

Meyer, I. H. (2003). Prejudice, social stress, and mental health in lesbian, gay, and bisexual populations: Conceptual issues and research evidence. *Psychological Bulletin, 129*(5), 674–697. https://doi.org/10.1037/0033-2909.129.5.674

Moscovici, S. (1963). Attitudes and opinions. *Annual Review of Psychology, 14*, 231–260. https://doi.org/10.1146/annurev.ps.14.020163.001311

Murray, S. O., & Roscoe, W. (Eds.). (1997). *Islamic homosexualities: Culture, history, and literature*. New York University Press.

Nardi, P. (1999). *Gay men's friendships: Invincible communities*. University of Chicago Press.

Orne, J. (2011). 'You will always have to "out" yourself': Reconsidering coming out through strategic outness. *Sexualities, 14*(6), 681–703. https://doi.org/10.1177/1363460711420462

Parwani, S., & Talukdar, A. K. (2024). Mental health of Indian LGBT+ community: Role of coping self-efficacy and social inclusion. *Mental Health and Social Inclusion, 28*(5), 561–573. https://doi.org/10.1108/MHSI-01-2023-0003

Siraj, A. (2011). Isolated, invisible, and in the closet: The life story of a Scottish Muslim lesbian. *Journal of Lesbian Studies, 15*(1), 99–121. https://doi.org/10.1080/10894160.2010.490503

Taylor, Y., & Snowdon, R. (Eds.). (2014). *Queering religion, religious queers.* Routledge.

Thöni, C., Eisner, L., & Hässler, T. (2024). Not straight enough, nor queer enough: Identity denial, stigmatization, and negative affect among bisexual and pansexual people. *Psychology of Sexual Orientation and Gender Diversity, 11*(2), 237–249. https://doi.org/10.1037/sgd0000606

Tillapaugh, D. (2013). Breaking down the "walls of a façade": The influence of compartmentalization on gay college males' meaning-making. *Culture, Society and Masculinities, 5*(2), 127–146. https://doi.org/10.3149/CSM.0502.127

Weeks, J. (2016). *Coming out: The emergence of LGBT identities in Britain from the 19th century to the present.* Quartet Books.

Weston, K. (1991). *Families we choose: Lesbians, gays, kinship.* Columbia University Press.

Williamson, I. R. (2000). Internalized homophobia and health issues affecting lesbians and gay men. *Health Education Research, 15*(1), 97–107. https://doi.org/10.1093/her/15.1.97

Wood, A. W., & Conley, A. H. (2014). Loss of religious or spiritual identities among the LGBT population. *Counseling and Values, 59*(1), 95–111. https://doi.org/10.1002/j.2161-007X.2014.00044.x

Yon-Leau, C., & Muñoz-Laboy, M. (2010). "I don't like to say that I'm anything": Sexuality politics and cultural critique among sexual-minority Latino youth. *Sexuality Research & Social Policy, 7*(2), 105–117. https://doi.org/10.1007/s13178-010-0009-y

4

Methodological Aspects of Researching Coming out

The Present Studies

There was a two-pronged methodological approach to the research described in this book. In the first stage of the research, written statements regarding either positive or negative coming out experiences to somebody significant were provided by a sample of 489 lesbian, gay, and bisexual (LGB) individuals and analyzed using qualitative thematic analysis. In the second stage of the research, interviews were conducted with a smaller sample of LGB individuals ($N = 22$) to examine in greater depth the themes that emerged from the first stage of the research. Data from the second stage of the research process were also analyzed using qualitative thematic analysis.

Stage 1: Written Accounts from Lesbian, Gay, and Bisexual People

Two experimental studies were originally conducted to examine the effects of recalling a coming out experience to a significant other for identity processes and psychological wellbeing. There were three inclusion criteria

R. Jaspal, *The Psychology of Coming Out*,
https://doi.org/10.1007/978-3-032-02599-9_4

for participating in the study: (1) being aged 18 or over; (2) self-identifying as lesbian, gay, or bisexual; and (3) having disclosed one's LGB identity to at least one person considered to be important (i.e., a significant other). In total, 489 LGB individuals were recruited on Prolific, an online participant recruitment platform, to participate in survey studies regarding the psychological effects of coming out. Table 4.1 provides a summary of the key demographic characteristics of the participant sample.

In both studies, participants were randomly allocated to one of two conditions: (1) to recall and describe a positive coming out experience to somebody significant, or (2) to recall and describe a negative coming out experience to somebody significant. Participants were asked to describe their experience in 5 or 6 sentences but no word limit was set on the online questionnaire. There was variation in the length of the accounts provided, ranging from a single sentence to 10 sentences. The two studies had two key objectives: first, to examine the causal role of recalling positive or negative coming out experiences on identity processes and psychological wellbeing which is described in other publications (Breakwell & Jaspal, 2022; Lopes & Jaspal, 2024) and, second, to provide a qualitative

Table 4.1 Socio-Demographic Characteristics of the Participant Sample (Study 1)

Variables	Categories	Frequency
Sex	Male	383
	Female	102
	Other	4
Ethnicity	White British	331
	Asian British	63
	Black British	19
	Mixed heritage	52
	Other	5
Sexual orientation	Lesbian	30
	Gay	352
	Bisexual	78
	Other	29
Relationship status	Single	252
	In a relationship	107
Education level	GCSE	57
	A-level	131
	Undergraduate degree	192
	Postgraduate degree	109

dataset to examine the most salient positive and negative features of LGB people's coming out experiences. This book is concerned with the latter.

LGB individuals of course come out repeatedly but not all coming out events are appended the same level of importance by the individual. This approach to data generation was deemed advantageous because participants were asked to home in on the most salient features of one significant coming out experience. Thus, they were instructed to be selective and, due to space constraints, to be focused in their identification of the key features of the experience. The exercise provided some scope for respondents to describe briefly the cognitive, affective, and behavioral aspects of these features. It is, for instance, shown in Chap. 5 that participants not only cited authenticity as a key positive feature of their coming out experience but also how this in turn shaped their feelings of self-esteem and other identity principles. Moreover, given the sensitive nature of the topic, it was deemed useful to complement the dyadic interview approach used in Stage 2 with an anonymized data generation approach that allowed individuals to share their experiences with reduced risk of social desirability bias. The qualitative data generated in those studies were extracted for qualitative thematic analysis.

Stage 2: Interviews with Lesbian, Gay, and Bisexual People

A sample of 22 LGB people was recruited to participate in an in-depth qualitative interview study focusing on the psychological aspects of coming out. As in Stage 1, there were three inclusion criteria for participating in the study: (1) being aged 18 or over; (2) self-identifying as lesbian, gay, or bisexual; and (3) having disclosed one's LGB identity to at least one person considered to be important. The first six participants were recruited from within the researcher's own social network and the remaining 16 participants were recruited using a snowball sampling strategy. Participants were interviewed virtually. Interviews lasted between 30 and 90 minutes. They were audio-recorded and then transcribed.

Participants were aged between 18 and 39 years ($M = 29.95$, $SD = 8.05$). Sixteen were resident in London and six in the English East Midlands.

All of them identified with the sex they were assigned at birth. Twelve participants were male, of whom eight identified as gay and four as bisexual, and 10 participants were female, of whom six identified as lesbians and four as bisexual. All the participants reported having come out as LGB to at least one person and 15 of the 22 participants focused on their experience of coming out to their parents in their interview accounts of coming out, although some of them also made reference to their experiences of coming out to other people.

The main purpose of the interview study was to triangulate the findings from Stage 1 of the research, to examine the emerging themes identified in Stage 1 in more detail, and to identify novel themes generated by participants themselves as they reflected upon their coming out experiences. The semi-structured interview schedule included questions that focused on a particularly important experience of coming out to somebody who mattered, feelings of authenticity, the impact of coming out on interpersonal relationships (including possible feelings of distance and loss), positive and negative reactions from people during the coming out process, and the impact of these reactions upon identity, emotion, and psychological wellbeing. As the interview schedule was semi-structured, it was sufficiently flexible so as to capture observations from participants that were not necessarily anticipated by the interviewer (or explicitly elicited in the interview schedule). For example, although the theme of microaggressions, gaslighting, and ghosting emerged in Stage 1, these were not explicitly asked about in Stage 2 but did emerge as key themes in interviewees' accounts when they were probed to discuss negative reactions to coming out. Given the brevity of the accounts provided in Stage 1, there was a focus on exploring in detail LGB people's experiences of coming out.

In view of the semi-structured nature of the interview schedule, some additional questions were iteratively introduced in order to probe further the issues that earlier participants had raised. Some interviewees introduced topics and issues that were not foreseen by the interviewer, which also prompted the use of questions not originally included in the interview schedule. As in Stage 1, the qualitative interview data were subjected to qualitative thematic analysis.

Doing the Analysis

Qualitative data can be subjected to many different types of analysis. Several approaches to the data analysis were considered, including content analysis, interpretative phenomenological analysis, narrative analysis, grounded theory, discourse analysis, and thematic analysis. All these approaches offer value but also have limitations.

The social constructionist commitment of discourse analysis provides important insight into the discursive constructions of people's experiences, often facilitating a fine-grained linguistic analysis of accounts, but its epistemological focus on social constructionism makes discourse analysis less useful for understanding cognition, affect, and behavior in relation to coming out (Burr, 2025; Jaspal, 2020). The focus on cognition was especially important in view of the objective to examine the impact of coming out for identity construction, development, and defense.

Conversely, interpretative phenomenological analysis is an inductive experiential methodology, foregrounding the individual's reported experiences on their own terms (Smith et al., 2021). However, the commitment of interpretative phenomenological analysis to phenomenology can preclude the a priori use of theory in the analysis. This was deemed disadvantageous given the significance of existing theories, such as the sexual identity development models (Chap. 2) and identity process theory and minority stress theory (Chap. 3), and the intention to use tenets of these theories as a template for interpreting LGB people's coming out experiences. Grounded theory has a focus upon the development of novel theory in the absence of existing theory (Charmaz, 2024). As this was not the objective of the studies, grounded theory was discarded as a possible methodology for examining the data.

Despite their limitations in relation to the present research, all these methodological approaches are useful for understanding LGB people's coming out experiences and would generate insight into different dimensions of it. For instance, discourse analysis could shed light on how coming out experiences are constructed linguistically to affirm particular identities in talk, while grounded theory might allow for the creation of a novel theory of coming out that addresses some of the limitations of the existing models outlined in Chap. 2. However, having considered all these approaches, the decision was taken to use qualitative thematic analysis through a realist epistemological lens.

Qualitative thematic analysis has been described as "method for identifying, analysing and reporting patterns (themes) within data" (Braun & Clarke, 2006, p. 78). This approach enables the analyst to identify key units of meaning in each coming out experience and to identify broader trends or patterns of meaning across different experiences. In contrast to discourse analysis and interpretative phenomenological analysis, thematic analysis is a flexible methodological approach that is not associated with any particular epistemology. Instead, it can incorporate elements of different epistemologies, such as social constructionism and realism. For instance, it is possible to use thematic analysis to derive themes that shed light on cognition, affect, and behavior in relation to coming out, while also examining the linguistic aspects of participants' constructions. This is how the methodology is used in this book.

The analytic steps for conducting thematic analysis described by Jaspal (2020) were followed. First, each data piece (i.e., each comment in Stage 1, and each interview transcript in Stage 2) was individually coded focusing upon the psychological aspects of each individual's coming out experience (including the cognitions and emotions that these generated) and the potential impact of coming out for identity processes. As such, the analysis actively drew upon elements of identity process theory and minority stress theory. Examples of preliminary codes included "sense of loss" and "perceived distance from significant others." Second, the preliminary codes were developed into themes, such as "emotional distance" and "loss of relationships." At the final step of the analysis, the themes were developed into master themes that represented key patterns of meaning across the entire dataset. These master themes, as well as selected quotes from the two datasets to exemplify them, are presented in Chaps. 5–9. Table 4.2 provides a summary of the master themes by chapter.

Table 4.2 Summary of Master Themes by Chapter

Chapter	Written Accounts	Interview Accounts
Deriving identity authenticity	(1) Deriving psychological wellbeing from authenticity (2) Authenticity and self-presentation (3) Authenticity and psychological safety	(1) Self-discovery and self-certainty (2) Being and feeling one's "true" self (3) The psychological functions of authenticity (4) The pitfalls of authenticity
Enhancing interpersonal relationships	(1) Continuation of existing relationships (2) Enhancement of existing relationships (3) Strengthening the family as a whole	(1) Relationship continuity (2) Providing a novel channel for open communication (3) Post-conflict trust and intimacy, and post-stress growth (4) Queering the family home
Rejection, emotional distance, and ambiguous loss	(1) Tension and loss in relationships (2) Emotional distance (3) Religion and culture as lenses for interpreting coming out	(1) Differentiating negative reactions from loss (2) The impact of loss for cognition, affect, and behavior (3) coping with rejection, emotional distance, and loss
Non-acknowledgement, invalidation, and silencing	(1) Non-acknowledgement (2) Invalidation (3) Silencing	(1) Playing a role (2) Undoing identity work (3) Threats to coherence
Psychological violence: Microaggressions, ghosting, and gaslighting	(1) Microaggressions (2) Ghosting (3) Gaslighting	(1) Microaggressions, self-esteem, and silence (2) Ghosting, uncertainty, and identity doubt (3) Gaslighting, identity doubt, and (re) construal

Triangulating the Findings

The purpose of including two sources of data, generated in different ways and from different participant samples, was to provide multi-faceted insights into the psychology of coming out. In Stage 1, a fairly large sample of LGB people provided brief written responses to a question eliciting information about either positive or negative coming out experiences and, in Stage 2, a smaller sample of LGB people described their positive and negative coming out experiences in greater detail and contextualized these experiences in previous ones as well as future expectations. Stage 1 was concerned primarily with identifying the key positive or negative aspects of a significant coming out experience to provide some structure to coming-out individuals' reported experiences. Stage 2 was concerned with the elaboration of key coming out experiences.

The topic of coming out is of course vast and LGB people come out numerous times, to different (and sometimes the same) people, and in different ways. The data generated in Stage 1 provided a means of orienting participants in Stage 2 toward particular themes that appeared to be significant for a fairly large sample of coming-out LGB individuals. This approach was advantageous because it allowed interviewees to describe the cognitive, affective, and behavioral dimensions of the issues presented (e.g., authenticity, psychological violence). Where these themes were less relevant to interviewees' experiences (in Stage 2), there was scope for other aspects of coming out to be discussed. Furthermore, as noted above, some themes identified in Stage 1, such as those concerning the specific forms of psychological violence experienced by coming-out individuals were not incorporated in the interview schedule used in Stage 2 but nonetheless emerged as key themes.

It is important to note that much of the empirical research reviewed in this book is quantitative and uses other research designs, such as cross-sectional correlational survey and experimental designs. The qualitative studies presented in the following chapters should be regarded against the backdrop of this existing largely quantitative research. They provide further qualitative depth and understanding of existing research and can help orient future research. For instance, Jaspal's (2025a, 2025b) model predicting degree of outness in LGB people postulates that social factors (e.g., exposure to minority stressors, the availability of social support) induce changes in identity (e.g., internalized homonegativity, sexual identity threat) that in turn determine decision-making regarding coming out. The findings of the studies reported in this book provide more nuanced qualitative insights into these social, intrapsychic, and behavioral factors underpinning coming out. No single empirical study should be viewed in isolation but rather in relation to the studies that have preceded it and as a basis for designing future studies.

Quality Assurance Issues

Qualitative research (and the analysis of data therein) is inherently subjective and, like research conducted using other methods, can be variable in quality. In order to ensure the quality of the qualitative analyses reported in this book, some quality assurance criteria were followed. Yardley (2000) has described four flexible principles as a guide for assessing the quality of a qualitative analysis.

- *Sensitivity to context.* It is good practice to reflect awareness of the dominant theories, previous empirical literature, and socio-cultural context in which the research has been conducted, and of participants' perspectives when undertaking the analysis.
- *Commitment and rigor* of the analysis. There should be in-depth engagement with the topic area through acknowledgement of previous research and how one's own research is positioned within that broader literature. The methodological approach must be clearly described and a strong rationale presented.
- *Transparency and coherence* of the data collection, analysis, and presentation of findings. It is important to present sufficient detail (i.e., extracts from the data) in order to demonstrate transparency and coherence. It is good practice to acknowledge the subjectivity that underpins qualitative research and to consider other possible interpretations.

- *Impact and importance* of the research questions and findings. The research questions must purport to fill a gap in knowledge that has been identified in the literature review. The research findings must have well-defined empirical, theoretical, and/or practical implications. For instance, the findings may challenge an existing theoretical paradigm or they may shed light on a given psychological phenomenon in a new population.

Ethical Aspects

Prior to commencing a research study, it is of course vital to think through the ethical aspects of conducting the research itself. As the studies reported in this book were being designed and conducted, the ethical dimension of the research was approached from a variety of perspectives. Three key ethical issues are especially noteworthy.

First, it was important to consider the possible broader implications of posing the specific research questions, as well as those of the findings. For instance, as highlighted in Chap. 1, there is a societal assumption (or social representation) that coming out is invariably a positive aspect of LGB identity development and, thus, coming out is socially valued while being "closeted" is stigmatized. How would the fact that the *negative* aspects of coming out were also being examined be understood by others? Similarly, how would the findings that there are some very negative consequences of coming out (e.g., exposure to microaggressions, gaslighting, and rejection) that possibly shape the attitudes, intentions, and behaviors of LGB people contemplating coming out in the future? Furthermore, it is seldom clear how one's research findings will be understood, used, and represented by others, such as in the media, by commentators on social media, and by political commentators. There is a risk that one's research, however well-intentioned the original aims, will be misunderstood, misused, or misrepresented. The truth is that the researcher can never control how their research findings will be interpreted, used, or represented by others but they can be clear in their own interpretation of the findings.

Second, the psychological wellbeing of the individuals who participated in Stage 1 was a key ethical consideration. Those who provided written accounts remained anonymous to the researcher since the accounts were provided as part of their participation in a quantitative survey study. All participants were asked to reflect upon either positive or negative experiences of coming out to somebody significant. Recalling a negative coming out experience could plausibly undermine psychological wellbeing by causing distress. Indeed, as outlined in Chaps. 7–9, participants did report distressing experiences, including those of psychological violence. This must be viewed against the backdrop of mental health inequalities experienced by LGB people compared to the general population which itself has been attributed to exposure to minority stressors (Frost & Meyer, 2023). Participants were provided with a detailed debrief sheet that included the contact details of support groups and healthcare services specializing in mental health issues.

Third, a specific ethical challenge associated with the interview study in the second stage regarding coming out experiences concerned the depth of the accounts that were elicited and, in many cases, provided by participants. After all, the aim of that study was to generate in-depth accounts that could be subjected to a fine-grained qualitative thematic analysis. This therefore required interviewees to recall and report in detail their experiences, cognitions, and emotions in relation to coming out. Not all of them were positive. Some reported behaving in ways they now regretted, thinking in ways that threatened their identities, and experiencing negative emotions. All this could be detrimental to psychological wellbeing. In contrast to the written accounts in which participants were asked to note cursorily their positive or negative experiences of coming out, in interviews they were asked to elaborate on their experiences and their responses were often probed further in an attempt to generate greater depth in their accounts. During the course of the research, some interviewees became visibly distressed as they recalled their experience. In these cases, the interview was paused and continued only when the participant felt comfortable to do so. As in Stage 1, all interviewees were provided with a detailed debrief sheet that included the details of support groups and healthcare services specializing in mental health support.

Limitations and Future Steps

The studies reported in this book have limitations that should be addressed in future research in this important area. Three are particularly noteworthy.

First, the studies both use a qualitative design and the analysis is inherently subjective. It is possible that other analysts would interpret the data differently, focus on different elements of participants' accounts, and reach different conclusions. It is necessary to triangulate the findings of these qualitative studies with quantitative data collected using other research design, such as cross-sectional survey and experimental designs.

Second, participants in both stages of the research were recruited in the United Kingdom and most of them self-identified as White British and reported being cisgendered. Future studies should build on these studies by exploring the coming out experiences of LGB people from other country contexts, from minority ethnic backgrounds, and with other gender identities. The recruitment of more diverse participant samples will help provide greater insight into the nature of coming out and its effects upon identity processes.

Third, it is important to note that the participants who shared their accounts of coming out in both stages of the research did so retrospectively. As a consequence, the data actually reflect the individual's current reflection of a past experience. It is thus not a "real-time" representation of their coming out experience but rather one viewed through the lens of the individual's current identity. Hindsight can enable the individual to reinterpret past experience in different ways. Changes that have occurred in identity since the past event can change the meanings that the individual now appends to that event. People may use coping strategies, such as reconstrual, to limit the degree of identity threat when recalling a threatening experience of coming out. In order to capture coming out in "real-time," it will be necessary to use other methods, such as diary study methods, that can chronicle the individual's experiences as the coming out event unfolds. This can provide insight into the contemporaneous cognitive, affective, and behavioral aspects of the coming out event.

Overview

This chapter outlines the wealth of methodological tools that can shed light on different psychological aspects of the coming out experience. The specific methodological aspects of the two studies reported in this book and the rationale for combining the two approaches are described. Qualitative thematic analysis was selected as an appropriate methodology for examining LGB people's written and interview accounts regarding their coming out experiences. It is noted that the studies reported in this book should not be viewed in isolation but rather in relation to the many empirical studies that have preceded them. Triangulation of these and previous studies can enable the analyst to build a fuller snapshot of the effects of coming out for identity processes. In the remaining chapters of this book, the results of the qualitative thematic analyses and their broader implications for understanding the psychology of coming out are described.

References

Braun, V., & Clarke, V. (2006). Using thematic analysis in psychology. *Qualitative Research in Psychology, 3*(2), 77–101. https://doi.org/10.1191/1478088706qp063oa

Breakwell, G. M., & Jaspal, R. (2022). Coming out, distress and identity threat in gay men in the United Kingdom. *Sexuality Research & Social Policy, 19*(3), 1166–1177. https://doi.org/10.1007/s13178-021-00608-4

Burr, V. (2025). *Social constructionism* (4th ed.). Routledge.

Charmaz, K. (2024). *Constructing grounded theory* (3rd ed.). Sage.

Frost, D. M., & Meyer, I. H. (2023). Minority stress theory: Application, critique, and continued relevance. *Current Opinion in Psychology, 51*, 101579. https://doi.org/10.1016/j.copsyc.2023.101579

Jaspal, R. (2020). Content analysis, thematic analysis and discourse analysis. In G. M. Breakwell, D. B. Wright, & J. Barnett (Eds.), *Research methods in psychology* (5th ed., pp. 285–312). Sage.

Jaspal, R. (2025a). A theoretical model for predicting outness in lesbian, gay and bisexual people: Minority stressors, social support, and identity processes. *Social Sciences, 14*(4), 207. https://doi.org/10.3390/socsci14040207

Jaspal, R. (2025b). Minority stressors, social connectedness and degree of outness in gay men: Data from two cross-sectional correlational studies in the United Kingdom. *Sexuality and Culture, 29*(3), 1318–1338. https://doi.org/10.1007/s12119-025-10325-4

Lopes, B., & Jaspal, R. (2024). Identity processes and psychological wellbeing upon recall of a significant "coming out" experience in lesbian, gay and bisexual people. *Journal of Homosexuality, 71*(1), 207–231. https://doi.org/10.1080/00918369.2022.2111536

Smith, J. A., Flowers, P., & Larkin, M. (2021). *Interpretative phenomenological analysis: Theory, method and research* (2nd ed.). Sage.

Yardley, L. (2000). Dilemmas in qualitative health research. *Psychology & Health, 15*(2), 215–228. https://doi.org/10.1080/08870440008400302

5

Deriving Identity Authenticity

What Is Identity Authenticity?

Identity authenticity has been defined as "the sense that one's life, both public and private, reflects one's real self" (George, 1998, p. 134) and being "true to oneself" is often presented as a key tenet of authenticity (Vannini & Franzese, 2008, p. 1621). Similarly, Varga (2014, p. 215) defines an authentic person as one that lives "in accordance with desires, motives, ideals or beliefs that are not only hers (as opposed to someone else's) but that also express who she really is." Hollier (2023) describes authenticity as being characterized by truth, confidence in one's identities, personal growth, freedom from the opinion of others, uninhibited connection with others, and resilience.

There are debates about the usefulness of the concept of authenticity since it is questionable whether a "real self" even exists and, if so, which component of the self is the focus given the multiplicity of identity and its continuous revision in response to change (e.g., Jaspal & Breakwell, 2014). As a psychological construct, identity authenticity is the individual's subjective perception about the congruence of their cognition, affect, and behavior with their "true self," whatever this may be and

R. Jaspal, *The Psychology of Coming Out*,
https://doi.org/10.1007/978-3-032-02599-9_5

however it is perceived and defined by the individual. In short, whether or not a true self exists is irrelevant—the key is that the individual believes they have a true self and that they recognize it and can act in accordance with their subjectively perceived true self.

Authenticity is socially valued, especially in the context of sexuality, and people are encouraged to live authentically, suggesting that inauthenticity is undesirable (Franzese, 2007; Guignon, 2008). The widespread social expectation and thus individual desire for authenticity are driven by essentialist perceptions of sexuality, that is, the notion that one has a "true" sexuality that is immutable (Fielder, 2015). Authenticity has also been conceptualized as a motivational force for self-enhancement, that is, as a means of deriving psychological wellbeing (George, 1998).

Authenticity and Wellbeing

There is now considerable research that shows that authenticity is associated with better mental health outcomes in lesbian, gay, and bisexual (LGB) people (Birichi, 2015; Levitt et al., 2016; Riggle et al., 2014; Villicana et al., 2016; Sutton, 2020) as well as many other social and psychological benefits, including self-efficacy (Russon & Schmidt, 2014). Rostosky et al. (2018) found that, compared to other positive identity variables, authenticity was the strongest predictor of all six domains of psychological wellbeing, namely autonomy, personal growth, environmental mastery, self-acceptance, purpose in life, and positive relations with others (see also Petrocchi et al., 2020).

There are many factors that can undermine a LGB person's feelings of authenticity, which in turn can have negative outcomes for their psychological wellbeing. The pressure to conform and feeling silenced by others can operate as impediments to authenticity. Valentine (2015) found that authenticity mediated the relationship between discrimination, including microaggressions, and psychological wellbeing. Similarly, in their study of 213 LGB people, Fredrick et al. (2020) found that the relationship between exposure to public stigma of their sexual identity and quality of life was mediated by feelings of authenticity. These results suggest that exposure to identity hazards, such as stigma, discrimination, concealment, and internalized homonegativity, undermine psychological wellbeing when they first curtail people's feelings of authenticity (e.g., Birichi, 2015).

Levitt et al. (2016) show in their grounded theory study of sexual minorities that minority stress arises from inauthenticity and decreased self-determination. They additionally note that people may feel pressured toward inauthenticity due to stigmatizing social representations of their sexuality and that inauthenticity may in turn thwart their sexual identity development. People nevertheless use creative strategies for navigating these powerful forces and for retaining a sense of wellbeing—not necessarily insisting on being authentic all the time but doing so strategically when the context is permissive of authenticity. A qualitative study of youth in a rural community in the Midwest of the United States found that the experience of hostility and threats of discrimination made it difficult for them to explore and express their sexualities openly but that many nevertheless sought out individuals and resources that could support them to do so (Rand & Paceley, 2022). This suggests that people generally strive for authenticity even in a relatively hostile social context.

This is unsurprising given the evidence that authenticity performs a protective role for psychological wellbeing. Brownfield et al. (2018) interviewed thirteen bisexual individuals about their coming out experiences. A significant theme in their narratives of coming out included the intrapersonal growth that they had experienced—most notably, the ability to live authentically which in turn was associated with better mental health. This is also observable in the workplace. In their study of 150 sexual minority employees, Fletcher and Everly (2021) found that the relationship between organizational lesbian, gay, bisexual, and transgender (LGBT) supportive practices and life satisfaction was mediated by feelings of authenticity. Similarly examining the impact of authenticity in the workplace, DuBois and Arena Jr. (2023) found that self-alienation (a proxy for inauthenticity) was associated with greater intention to leave the organization through the mediator of reduced affective commitment. Thus, bisexuals who felt they could not be themselves in turn reported lower affective commitment to the organization and thus a proclivity to leave the organization. Gardner and Prasad (2022) found that the relationship between authentic expression and positive organizational outcomes (i.e., commitment and involvement) was moderated by perceived psychological safety. In other words, authenticity seems to have beneficial outcomes only when people feel psychologically safe in their social context.

Psychological safety may be derived through a variety of means—through supportive practices and norms in the workplace, as well as affirmative interpersonal relationships with others. Indeed, in their study of same-gender couples, Chen et al. (2024) found that individuals' identity authenticity was positively related to their sense of relationship satisfaction only when their partner had low levels of internalized homonegativity. Furthermore, internalized homonegativity—itself a product of stigmatizing social representations of one's sexuality—was inversely associated with feelings of identity authenticity.

Outness and Authenticity

The relationship between outness and authenticity is complex. People of course derive authenticity from many different sources and on the basis of different elements of identity. Sexuality is just one of them. Fletcher and Everly (2021) found that the relationship between coming out and authenticity was moderated by identity centrality, suggesting that coming out is more conducive to feelings of authenticity when people actually view their sexuality as being more central to their identity. Conversely, it could be surmised that those LGB people who do not view their sexuality as especially central to their identity would be less reliant upon being out in order to derive authenticity.

Outness has been conceptualized in many different ways. For instance, Brownfield and Brown (2022) conceptualize outness in terms of a proximal minority stressor, since it can expose the individual to stigma, rejection, and discrimination, while Jaspal and Breakwell (2022) conceptualize it as a positive coping strategy that can facilitate feelings of validation and authenticity. In other words, some LGB people may decide to come out in the pursuit of validation and affirmation of their sexuality, especially when they are habitually exposed to negative social representations of it.

The relationships between outness, concealment, authenticity, and psychological wellbeing outcomes are complex.

In their study of 373 LGB participants, Riggle et al. (2017) found that increased outness was associated with lower psychological wellbeing, while LGB-specific concealment and feelings of authenticity were positively associated with psychological wellbeing outcomes. Several points are noteworthy. First, it may be possible to derive feelings of authenticity without being out to everybody—people are sometimes selective in whom they tell and the extent to which they tell them about their sexuality. Second, in some contexts, being more out may actually lead to increased exposure to identity hazards, such as discrimination. Third, concealing one's sexual identity is generally associated with decreased wellbeing but, in some cases, this may be the lesser of two evils. Clearly, all this will depend upon social context. In a hostile social context in which homonegativity is rife, being out may be more psychologically challenging than gratifying.

Yet, it does appear that the desire to be authentic motivates at least some LGB people to come out. In their discourse analysis study, Holt and Griffin (2003) showed that their lesbian and gay participants strove to seek spaces in which they could derive a sense of authenticity in relation to their lesbian and gay identities and that they did so on the "gay scene." Thus, they proactively sought spaces in which they could be out and authentic. This is consistent with the observation that coming out can be a coping strategy especially in the face of social censure of one's sexuality (Jaspal & Breakwell, 2022). This desire to be out could be attributed to the distress reported by LGB people when they feel compelled to conceal their identity. Indeed, in semi-structured interviews with 18 gay men, Williams (2023) found a theme of self-alienation from one's authentic self which arose when individuals used the "false self" strategy to prevent feelings of rejection due to homonegativity. However, by fostering positive social interaction with other gay men (through friendship), they could construct a more authentic sense of self. Furthermore, as noted in Chap. 1, there does appear to be social pressure to be out and authentic. For instance, Lovelock (2019) analyzed 35 coming out videos on YouTube and found a strong theme of making public an authentic "truth" of one's identity which constructed coming out as socially normative and, by implication, sexual identity concealment as problematic.

Authenticity often competes with the need for social approval from others (Goffman, 1967). Living authentically may expose the individual to social disapproval, especially if the identity element in question is socially stigmatized, as sexuality often is. People of course vary in the extent to which they feel the need for social approval, but it has been shown that perceiving the need for social approval is negatively associated with living authentically (Franzese, 2007). People may engage in impression management, which amounts to strategic self-presentation in the face of anticipated social disapproval and as a means of protecting identity from threat (Goffman, 1963; Leary & Kowalski, 1990; Roth et al., 1986). As some commentators focus on behavior in the enactment of authenticity, it is sometimes assumed that those who engage in impression management or passing—feigning an identity that they do not actually hold—tend to derive lower levels of identity authenticity. This is not necessarily the case. After all, an individual may actually have high levels of internal authenticity and, at the psychological level, understand what they want from life, and know who they are but, for self-protection, conceal this identity from others in particular social contexts (Cartwright et al., 2023).

Written Accounts from Lesbian, Gay, and Bisexual People

In this section, the following three themes arising from the thematic analysis of written accounts from LGB people are reported: (1) deriving psychological wellbeing from authenticity; (2) authenticity and self-presentation; and (3) authenticity and psychological safety.

Deriving Psychological Wellbeing from Authenticity

For some LGB people, life prior to coming out is characterized by inauthenticity. Some feel unable to express their "true" selves and thus obliged to present themselves inauthentically. Some must feign heterosexuality to evade social censure. Some live in fear. When participants were asked to recount a positive coming out experience, the theme of identity authenticity was prominent in their accounts. Most participants described the positive feelings of authenticity that they derived upon coming out to someone who mattered to them:

> With family and friends I had to just make these socially correct comments about how fit a girl is when it did nothing for me. When I came out, that all stopped (thank God) and I could at least stop pretending and just say who I really like or not say anything at all because I didn't feel the pressure.

> I was living a lie and was petrified I was going to get found out but that all went away once my parents knew. They made me think I can just be myself and that was the best thing of all. I was just 16 but it was the best gift they'd given me. I felt like I could do what it takes to get on in life now.

> Suddenly the lying all stopped and I could just be me. That felt really good. I felt quite validated by it all like I didn't have to lie anymore. Like a weight off my shoulders.

In their accounts, respondents contrasted their past feelings and experiences of inauthenticity with the newfound sense of authenticity they were afforded upon coming out. There were references to passing, that is, feigning heterosexuality, in order to avoid social stigma and to derive feelings of acceptance and inclusion. Individuals reported feeling pressured to be dishonest: "living a lie." The feelings of acceptance and inclusion that passing facilitated was clearly at odds with the feelings of authenticity that they also sought. Individuals may opt for inauthenticity in order to avoid stigma from significant others. By addressing one psychological challenge (a potential threat to self-esteem), they unwittingly allowed another to develop, that is, decreased authenticity. As seen in the extracts above, participants wished to "just be myself" and to "just be me." There was some evidence that this actually provided feelings of self-esteem ("that felt really good"), validation, and also self-efficacy, as one individual stated that they could now "do what it takes to get on in life." Others reflected on the meanings of authenticity for them:

> Pretty much everything remained the same, apart from the fact I can be more open about who I am. I've been able to express myself a lot more, but everyone treats me the same.

> It was scary but the thing that stayed consistent was respectful boundary setting for themselves and me. I would know limits to conversations with some people. I was fortunate enough to have a few people that I could be fully open and be myself.

Authenticity was defined by some individuals as being "more open about who I am" and the ability to "express myself a lot more" regardless of their actual relationship with other people. For them, authenticity consisted of the ability to be, and express, themselves. It is noteworthy that some people acknowledged that this sense of authenticity was not dependent upon coming out to everyone or even having the ability to discuss with them openly their sexuality but rather their own perceived ability to be "fully open" with particular individuals. As shown in the extracts above, there was awareness of the "limits to conversations with some people," but this did not necessarily compromise feelings of authenticity as individuals resourcefully managed how and with whom they could be authentic. The method for deriving authenticity was not the same across all contexts and relationships—in some, it was possible to acknowledge but not discuss openly their sexual identity while in others this was an important determinant of feeling authentic. Feelings of authenticity were also associated with self-enhancement and, in particular, self-confidence:

> Luckily my parents and friends have always supported me even if at the beginning they were incredulous of my homosexuality and this gave me more self-confidence.

> My parents made me feel like a whole person when I came out and they encourage me to be myself.

> Telling my parents was scary—not going to lie—but they made me feel quite whole, like all my life now just fit together. I was a more confident person and loved myself more when I told them.

These accounts converge in demonstrating the positive psychological functions that can be performed by authenticity when LGB people come out. Participants noted that parental support to be authentic in turn provided them with greater self-confidence, made them "feel like a whole person," and made them believe that their life "now just fit together." It appears that authenticity can generate feelings of psychological coherence, that is, the perception that elements of identity are coherent and consistent (Jaspal & Cinnirella, 2010). This itself is contingent upon support, encouragement, and validation from significant others (most notably, one's parents) upon coming out. It was clear from participants' written accounts that self-presentation and, specifically, the ability to present themselves in ways deemed to be consistent with their "inner" or "true" self were key to deriving feelings of authenticity.

Authenticity and Self-Presentation

Given their fear of stigmatization and, in some cases, rejection, individuals had previously felt pressured to conceal their identity and to pass as heterosexual—to achieve this they had to self-present and behave in particular ways. Yet, coming out provided some psychological respite as it finally enabled them to align their self-presentation with their true identity:

> My mum had always told me to cut my hair short and my dad made comments about it but when they understood they started encouraging me just to buy stuff for my hair. I felt like they really accepted me and I could just be who I really am. That was my best coming out really.

> Coming out to my parents was like breaking free. I wore my rainbow flag t-shirt when I sat them down. It had always been hidden away but out it came and on it went. I broke free when I came out and that felt good and validating.

> I could just relax for the first time in my life when my mum and dad just asked me and I told them. I could stop hiding stuff showing I'm gay, like internet history. I didn't need to hide myself.

Respondents described a range of experiences and behaviors, such as their parents' disapproval of particular hairstyles and the perceived need to conceal certain items of clothing and their Internet browser history, in order to prevent involuntary disclosure of their sexuality. These tenets and activities may seem relatively trivial to the outside observer but to individuals themselves they constituted important markers of their sexual identity. They were fearful of being discovered. However, when they came out, they felt empowered to self-present in ways that aligned with their true identity.

Powerful language was used to describe the feelings of authenticity that this facilitated. Participants described this in terms of "breaking free," the ability to "just be who I really am," and no longer needing "to hide myself." The ensuing feelings of authenticity, following significant periods of inauthenticity, provided self-enhancement ("that felt good") as well as a sense of validation from significant others. It is noteworthy that coming out can facilitate not only feelings of authenticity in the present moment but also create a context for continued authenticity in the long term. One participant reported that their hairstyle was not only accepted by their parents but that they now felt encouraged to maintain it. Crucially, individuals felt empowered to be authentic because they perceived a sense of psychological safety from people who mattered to them.

Authenticity and Psychological Safety

For some, a favorable reaction to coming out signaled to them that they now possessed a "safe space" in which they could be themselves and thus derive feelings of authenticity. This did not necessarily mean that they could always be authentic in every context but rather that there now existed some contexts involving people who mattered to them in which they could self-present in ways that felt authentic to them:

> Home was scary before coming out but when my parents listened and accepted me I felt like it became a safe space for me to be me.

> I am living my best life after telling my dad (my mum died a few years ago). Home is like a safe space for me. I can tell him but there's no pressure. Not

> to tell him anything or anyone. He just sits there and lets me talk. I can just be my true self and not who other people want me to be.

> My best friend didn't tell nobody and didn't force me to tell nobody. I felt really confident and just OK with being myself around her.

LGB people sometimes report feeling pressured to conform to heteronormative norms which could jeopardize their own identity authenticity. In these extracts, it appears that liberation from those coercive norms and the ability to reveal however much of one's identity that one wishes to collectively serve to bolster feelings of authenticity. In addition to their characterization of the home as a safe space, some participants noted that they now felt "no pressure." Another form of societal pressure—namely to come out publicly as LGB and to be open about one's sexuality—was also alluded to in the extracts.

Yet, the ability to choose when to come out, to whom, and to what extent also enhanced authenticity and broader wellbeing. Participants described their relief in no longer feeling pressured to discuss aspects of their sexuality that they did not wish to discuss. Moreover, they felt safe in the knowledge that their sexuality would not be involuntarily disclosed to others. Indeed, one participant's best friend did not disclose her sexuality to others (or "out" her) and she also did not feel obliged to tell anyone else. The key point is that, for some LGB people, the prospect of losing control over disclosure is deeply threatening and can lead them to fear and thus avoid coming out even to significant others. Having the latitude to determine one's own identity and future is key to the derivation of authenticity.

Coming out to a supportive significant other may not only provide feelings of authenticity but also put into place a social psychological infrastructure for continuing to derive such feelings:

> I came out to my mum and she has never treated me different. In fact she has been the only member of my family that I have had the courage to come out to so far. I am still in the early stages of telling everyone but I don't feel that it should be a big deal. My mother often encourages me to come out to everyone and offers me her full support.

> I told my aunt and uncle who brought me up. They told me they didn't bring me up to hide but to be proud of who I am and where I am and it meant a lot to me. I always think about them when I'm tempted to pretend or tell a lie about who I am and I don't do it. I'm just me.

These participants referred to the positive psychological impact of their coming out experiences, which in turn generated greater confidence to continue to come out to others. Indeed, some acknowledged finding it difficult to come out to family members, electing only to come out to particular individuals (e.g., one's mother). However, the positive experience of doing so engendered the belief that coming out to others was possible and could have favorable consequences. In other words, one positive coming out experience may provide greater confidence for coming out to others in the future.

Across both testimonies, it was clear that being encouraged to share one's identity with others, in addition to feeling supported to do so, was a key underpinning of the authenticity people derived upon coming out to someone significant. This should be contrasted with the perception that one's significant others may apparently accept one's sexuality but prefer that the dissemination and circulation of this information be limited. Indeed, some LGB people who come out report that their significant others ask them not to come out to other family members in order to avoid stigma (see Chap. 8). Furthermore, as noted above, some participants noted that the acceptance, support, and encouragement they obtained from significant others when they came out to them had a lasting impact on their identity authenticity—one participant reported thinking of them when feeling "tempted to pretend or lie about who I am."

The theme of allyship was prominent in LGB people's written accounts of coming out. For some participants, their significant others not only accepted their sexuality when they came out but also became supporters and advocates for LGB people:

> I was feeling really afraid but my mum just said I'm still her son and this doesn't change anything and she was proud that I'm being true to myself. It made me feel true to myself too. She's been a real ally as in full 180 degrees turn from where she was.

> My mum said the nicest thing. She said sorry for all the microaggressions because she didn't know. She doesn't stand for any shit now so I just feel not just I am who I am but I love myself more and owe this to her. She just sticks up for me.

> My sister is like my rock now. I could finally be myself around her and just tell her who I'm meeting (a girl) and if anyone said something bad about lesbians, she would be onto them straight away. She's an LGBT ally now.

A significant impediment to authenticity is one's own internalized homonegativity which tends to stem from stigma that one encounters in social contexts, especially from significant others. Yet, this barrier may be removed when LGB people encounter identity acceptance and validation from significant others. In short, to be told that one is worthy and loveable, especially when fearing stigma and rejection, bolsters self-esteem. As noted above, respondents' significant others provided encouragement to be authentic and even made amends for previous microaggressions not only by apologizing but also through their allyship. More specifically, rather than being a bystander to homonegativity, the proactive intervention of significant others to defend LGB identities could provide feelings of acceptance and validation. This is possibly why one of the participants described their significant other as "my rock."

Interview Accounts from Lesbian, Gay, and Bisexual People

In this section, the following four themes arising from the thematic analysis of the interview accounts from LGB people are described: (1) self-discovery and self-certainty; (2) being and feeling one's "true" self; (3) the psychological functions of authenticity; and (4) the pitfalls of authenticity.

Self-Discovery and Self-Certainty

In interviews, all participants made reference to the intrapsychic dimension of coming out, that is, their own recognition of their sexual orientation and its construction as an identity, in addition to the interpersonal dimension of sharing their sexual identity with other people. For several individuals, coming out at an intrapsychic level entailed a process of self-discovery and, in some cases, one of overcoming doubts about their sexuality:

> First you come out to yourself then maybe, just maybe you decide to come out to other people but the two aren't necessarily related for me. I'm talking about my case. It wasn't for me totally related. I've known and accepted me for me and so I've come out to myself. But now I feel more sure of myself and there's no doubt in my head, even the smallest doubt. It's weird. (Sam, gay man)

Coming out enabled Sam to derive greater feelings of certainty about his gay identity and to overcome any doubts that he had previously had about it. Like Sam, others noted that they had been aware of their sexuality for a considerable period of time. However, exposure to negative social representations of their sexuality, especially from other people who were unaware of it, generated discomfort and, in some cases, doubts. For some, this was wishful thinking—some came to believe that maybe they were not really LGB but that this was a phase or that they were confused or curious. Yet, as Sam noted, coming out—at both intrapsychic and interpersonal levels—marked important identity milestones, primarily because they were now in a position to derive certainty about who they were. They now felt more secure in their sexual identities. For some, doubts about their sexuality were assuaged by coming out:

> It [coming out] just gave me that feeling of now knowing and never doubting because before then I'd been like "yeah, maybe I'm a lesbian or maybe I'm not, maybe I'm straight." I was just lying to myself, forget everyone else. I was telling myself what basically other people wanted to hear, that I was straight. Well, no, I'm not and that's what coming out is really. It's knowing and then telling people that you know and they aren't going to change you now. All of this like made it seem more real and I felt more real, more true, as a person. (Sarah, lesbian woman)

Sarah also highlighted the doubts that she previously had in relation to her sexuality, which she attributed to her desire to conform socially. Like Sarah, several interviewees noted that they were not only concealing their sexuality from other people but from themselves: "I was just lying to myself." Due to negative social representations of their sexuality, some individuals themselves came to internalize negative beliefs about being LGB. Identity process theory refers to denial as a possible strategy for assuaging real or potential threats to identity—this appeared to be the strategy employed by some of those who were struggling to retain a positive sense of identity in the face of social pressures. Yet, coming out appeared to offer an alternative coping strategy: "now knowing and never doubting," that is, recognition of their sexual identity. Crucially, Sarah and others framed this process of self-discovery as a landmark in their lives which definitively put an end to the self-doubt that had previously besieged their sense of identity. This acceptance strategy of self-recognition replaced the previous deflection strategy of denial employed by some and itself generated feelings of authenticity: "I felt more real, more true, as a person."

Individuals clearly differentiated between coming out as intrapsychic and interpersonal processes. Coming out to oneself (i.e., at the intrapsychic level) appeared to be especially significant:

> You know, I consider myself out, my folks know, my close friends know but that doesn't mean I tell everyone. Sometimes I just stay quiet and don't say anything and sometimes—yeah, it's true—I lie about it [his sexuality] but it doesn't bother me personally because I know and the ones I love most know though strictly speaking that is not true. My grandparents don't know and I love them but I know. That's what matters. (James, bisexual man)

> I feel true to myself even if I'm not 100% true to everyone I meet. You got to look after your own safety and mental health and sometimes it just isn't a good call to blurt it out. Like when I go to Church, I don't tell the pastor that I'm a lesbian. It would hurt my mum even though she accepts me fully but that doesn't change how I feel about myself and I personally couldn't care less about what the pastor thinks. (Sally, lesbian woman)

James, a bisexual man, thoughtfully reflected upon the extent of his outness and noted that not all his loved ones were aware of his sexual identity. This was not deemed to be problematic since, for him, his own awareness of his sexuality was of primary importance. Similarly, Sally contrasted her intrapsychic authenticity ("I feel true to myself") with her self-presentation to others ("I'm not 100% true to everyone I meet"). She clearly prioritized intrapsychic authenticity over authentic self-presentation to others because the latter must be considered in the broader context of other people's beliefs, attitudes, and behaviors. Indeed, Sally and other interviewees referred to interpersonal and institutional constraints on authentic self-presentation. As a practicing Christian, Sally did not deem it beneficial for her safety or mental health to disclose her lesbian identity to her pastor nor to her mother with whom she had a positive relationship.

Crucially, individuals deemed it possible to compartmentalize their self-presentation to others—even significant others—and their own intrapsychic authenticity. Indeed, as Sally noted, her "inauthentic" self-presentation to others did not necessarily undermine her own intrapsychic authenticity. Various strategies were employed to do this—Sally appeared to reduce the significance of the pastor's beliefs about lesbians which reflected the coping strategy of negativism, that is, "the state of mind which one is in when one feels a desire or a compulsion to act *against* the requirements or pressures from some external source" (Apter, 1983, p. 79). She also noted that, although her mother was unaware of her lesbian identity, she was otherwise "fully" accepting of her.

James, Sally, and others contrasted their process of self-discovery with the doubts they had previously experienced in relation to their sexuality. This was described by some as traumatic:

> The biggest shame I felt was lying to myself, not anyone else, and I did it for years. (Chris, gay man)

> Not being true to yourself especially about something so basic and intrinsic like your sexuality is a trauma that sort of stays with you but it gets better because you feel all the more proud of yourself when you do admit it to yourself without making excuses. (Jamie, bisexual woman)

Doubting his identity was deemed by Chris to be the most significant source of shame he had felt in his life while for Jamie this was an enduring trauma despite having now assimilated and accommodated her bisexual identity. Several participants who referred to this early sense of self-doubt used emotive, self-castigating language, such as "lying to myself" and "not being true to yourself." They were clearly referring to the significance of authenticity at the intrapsychic level. Crucially, the process of coming to terms with their sexuality at the intrapsychic level was deemed to be the starting point, enabling them subsequently to share this information with other people. In short, being and feeling one's "true" self was a key step in the coming out process.

Being and Feeling One's "True" Self

There was a clear sense among interviewees that self-disclosure or sharing their sexuality with significant others reinforced the process of being and feeling their "true" self, suggesting a reciprocal relationship between self-discovery and self-disclosure to others.

> Coming out to me was like "this is me, the real me, not the fake me" and I was basically saying this to the two most important people in my life who supposedly knew me and brought me up as a child, gave me my name, fed me, clothed me. Like at last they were meeting the "real me" and I can't put this into words, the feeling it gave me. (Sally, lesbian woman)

Sally contrasted her "true" self with the "fake me" which she had felt compelled to exhibit prior to coming out. Her coming out experience was especially significant at the psychological level because it enabled her to present her "true" self to the most significant people in her life, namely her parents. This is an important point because, for Sally and several others, coming out was not about being authentic to everybody but rather to those individuals who really mattered. As seen across other extracts presented in this chapter, the pressure to be inauthentic and, in some cases, to be dishonest about one's identity was psychologically challenging. It often undermined people's sense of self-esteem. Indeed, Sally implied that it was psychologically taxing to be inauthentic to people who had played such an important role in her upbringing and noted that her current ability to show her true self was especially positive for her. The psychological burden of hiding was echoed by others in the participant sample:

> Hiding yourself is tiring. It's almost as bad as the direct attacks on your sexuality. It's like being invisible. It feels good to just be yourself, your true self. I felt like I was in a way complicit in the homophobia I got from homophobes, you know, by denying who I really am. (Jim, bisexual man)

Jim likened the experience of "hiding yourself" to that of homonegativity. For him, hiding oneself and therefore "being invisible" was comparable to being victimized due to one's sexuality. He also constructed concealment of his sexuality and passing as heterosexual as acts of complicity in homonegativity as he felt that homonegativity was vindicated by his silence. He and other participants suggested that deriving authenticity—by coming out to significant others—was beneficial for self-esteem. All this demonstrates the importance not only of reducing homonegativity but of proactively creating spaces in which LGB people feel comfortable sharing their identity with others and especially significant others.

Joe noted the significance of coming out in view of prior experiences of homonegativity and the more general challenges associated with sexual identity concealment:

> I've had a lot of bad reactions to coming out before and it does make you depressed and a bit scared actually but what really stands out for me more than anything else is the one great experience of coming out to someone who really mattered a lot to me and that overshadows all the bad stuff. All the insults, bullying, I just felt like "yeah, I can confront that head-on and take the bull by the horns" and that's why being true to yourself, to someone you don't want to lie to does for you. (Joe, gay man)

> Being true to myself sort of gave my life a bit more meaning. I just saw my life as being more logical. As in "this is who I am" and not just hiding anymore. (Jen, lesbian woman)

Joe acknowledged the negative emotions and state of depression that he had experienced in response to unfavorable reactions to his sexuality. However, in his view, a single positive experience of coming out to someone significant could supersede all these negative prior experiences of homonegativity, such as verbal attacks and bullying behaviors. In other words, a positive coming out experience was by far more meaningful and more powerful than his many negative prior experiences. His account suggested that "being true" not only to himself but also to significant others provided feelings of self-efficacy, that is, feelings of competence and control. Similarly, Jen's account indicated that "not just hiding anymore" imbued her life with a greater sense of meaning and logic, suggesting greater identity continuity.

An important unifying thread throughout participants' accounts was the dual relation between intrapsychic authenticity and interpersonal authenticity (involving somebody significant, such as a parent). Kim and Michael highlighted their positive feelings upon coming out to somebody who mattered:

> To me, it was just like a feeling of being safe and feeling understood and seeing the real me and not just what they always hoped for in a daughter. You know what I mean, marrying a guy and having kids and whatnot. It was special to feel understood as a real person. (Kim, bisexual woman)

> My dad said to me "well, son, you're not the only one, there are lots of your kind around so you're not alone." For a manly man like him to say that to me, it was out of this world. I thought I could really be accepted and just be seen as me and not just as a gay guy or as a "poof" like he used to say before. (Michael, gay man)

For both Kim and Michael, a significant underpinning of their authenticity was the recognition that they received from significant others (in their case, their parents) upon coming out to them. Kim valued "feeling understood" and that her mother now saw her "real" identity as a bisexual woman, putting aside her own prior aspirations for her daughter. Michael valued feeling accepted as well as "being seen as me" rather than primarily as a gay man. In both cases, the positive reaction to coming out was largely unexpected—Kim's mother had long hoped for a heterosexual daughter and Michael's father ("a manly man") had previously made derogatory remarks about gay people. Participants deeply valued their parents' ability to put aside their own expectations, aspirations, and even beliefs in order to accommodate their sexuality and, in Michael's case, to reassure him. His father was clearly attempting to perform a supportive pastoral role and did so in his own way. These experiences appeared to augment the authenticity that LGB people so often seek when coming out.

The Psychological Functions of Authenticity

It has been shown throughout this chapter that the derivation of authenticity is clearly one motivating factor for coming out as LGB. In most cases, individuals described a sense of relief upon becoming "true" to themselves. They often did so even when the reaction that they had hoped for did not materialize. Participants' accounts revealed some of the psychological functions of authenticity itself:

> I told someone I love a lot about me and I was bringing the inside out. I mean, I was being myself and just let myself go, sharing that with the person most important to me so they could see me as I see myself. That was a special moment because I was feeling that finally this person knows me, the real me that loves them. (Julie, lesbian woman)

Julie's account of coming out to her mother demonstrated one of the significant benefits of interpersonal authenticity: she could finally reveal the "real me" to someone who mattered to her, to somebody she loved. She described this metaphorically as "bringing the inside out," suggesting that the "real me" or "the inside" had previously been concealed. Julie appeared to distinguish between the "real me" and another facet of the self which was not explicitly mentioned. It was the "real me" that was capable of valuing (and loving) her significant others. This was described as a mechanism of strengthening her relationship with her mother who finally came to know her when she came out. (The positive impact of coming out for interpersonal relationships is the focus of Chap. 6.)

Interpersonal authenticity clearly had implications for psychological wellbeing at the intrapsychic level:

> When I came out to her [his mother] I held my breath. I actually remember that and her face just told me she accepted me for who I am. I felt real for once and, yes, it felt good. I felt like someone of worth and could stop feeling guilty all the same. My God, all that shame, it was basically disabling. It had a disabling effect but by first being myself, I could learn to love myself. That's what coming out did for me. (Bill, gay man)

For Bill, "feeling real" (intrapsychic authenticity) appeared to enhance feelings of self-esteem. Indeed, Bill noted that by coming out he was now in a position to value himself and to view himself as "someone of worth." Furthermore, by coming out and being authentic, he felt liberated from the negative emotional experience of guilt associated with the concealment of his sexual identity from significant others. He and others in the sample described feelings of guilt due to the need not only to conceal their true self but also to present an inauthentic version of the self, that is, to pass as heterosexual.

> Coming out for the first time really isn't an easy thing. Quite the opposite. The fear, the shame, all that eats you up and that's why a lot of people try to commit suicide or self-harm. I didn't but it did cross my mind because I was suffering quite a lot about being bisexual. But coming out and realizing you're still alive and still loved, it gives you power. It's like an energy that gets you through the day. Then the next time I did it, it was uncomfortable but better and it just gets better and better and better. You can actually do things and you start to believe in yourself more. (Mike, bisexual man)

All the interviewees acknowledged the challenging dimension of coming out. This carried with it an element of risk since individuals were not always certain of the reaction that coming out would elicit from others, especially from valued others. Like Bill, Mike experienced a variety of negative emotions, including fear and shame, which he linked to suicidal ideation. He reported suffering due to the need to conceal his bisexual identity. This was clearly psychologically distressing for many of those who disclosed such experiences of enforced inauthenticity. Yet, coming out enabled him to feel "alive" and "still loved," which suggested that authenticity was conducive to feelings of self-esteem. Moreover, coming out reportedly provided feelings of power and "energy that gets you through the day," indicating that there were also positive implications for his sense of self-efficacy. He reported feeling empowered to overcome the discomfort associated with coming out. In short, the positive coming out experience that he described in turn enabled him to come out again and again. By coming out and being authentic, Mike derived greater self-esteem and self-efficacy. Others echoed these positive outcomes of authenticity for identity:

> I would describe my mum's reaction as compassionate. She showed compassion and understood me. When someone does that, it makes you think "here this person is loving me and I hate myself. What's all that about?" So that compassion made me more compassionate toward myself too. It is sort of a positive circle. They love you, so you love yourself. (Karen, bisexual woman)

As noted above, interpersonal authenticity had positive outcomes for intrapsychic authenticity and for other identity principles at the intrapsychic level. For Karen, the compassion that she encountered from her mother when she came out as bisexual enabled her to reflect upon her own self-image. She reported low self-esteem prior to coming out ("I hated myself") but, upon coming out to her mother and encountering a compassionate response from a person who mattered to her, she projected this compassion onto her own self-conception. Karen reportedly learned to be more compassionate toward herself and thus build her own feelings of self-esteem. Crucially, her account and those of several others suggested that one's self-conception is, at least in part, contingent upon the conception that others have of one. Karen alluded to a reciprocal relationship between compassion from significant others and compassion toward herself. She reported her newfound ability to love herself, that is, to derive self-esteem, as did others:

> Hiding and lying and pretending and sneaking about, all that is really tiring. I realized I didn't have time to think about myself or what I felt about myself. I didn't have a second because I was just worrying all the time. The minute I told my parents and they opened up to me, it was incredible. Like a massive weight off my shoulders and I could give myself some self-care and focus on myself and feel good about myself. Coming out was the best decision I ever made, that's for sure. (Bill, gay man)

Bill contrasted the psychological burden of concealing his sexual identity from others with the positive interpersonal and intrapsychic aspects of coming out to his parents. Indeed, individuals who felt compelled to hide and pass as heterosexual generally reported anxiety and limited self-care behaviors. They simply did not feel that they had the time or opportunity to focus on their own wellbeing precisely because they were so fixated on passing. Bill described his coming out experience not only in terms of disclosing his sexuality but also in terms of his parents' reaction of "opening up" to him. As discussed in Chap. 6, this could have favorable outcomes for the quality of one's relationships with significant others. Yet, for Bill, the primary benefit of his coming out was his ability to focus on himself, engage in self-care behaviors, and, consequently, to derive feelings of self-esteem. For Jim, being interpersonally authentic appeared to be beneficial for his sense of continuity:

> I could finally be myself around people and it was like my acting or like my way of being around people was more, like it fitted more with how I always was, like the real me. It's hard to explain, almost like the inside and the outside were now overlapping and not like two different people. (Jim, bisexual man)

As indicated by several interviewees, the need for sexual identity concealment led to a rupture in continuity between the "real" self and the version of the self presented to other people. Interpersonal authenticity—the ability to exhibit the true self to other people—appeared to restore feelings of continuity. In spite of the benefits of authenticity for self-esteem, self-efficacy, and continuity, the process of deriving authenticity also presented some challenges for identity.

The Pitfalls of Authenticity

Authenticity is often framed in positive terms, that is, as something that one aspires to achieve (Vannini & Franzese, 2008). Authenticity is celebrated when it is achieved. People who lack authenticity are stigmatized. It has been shown in this chapter that authenticity can indeed have positive outcomes for identity processes and psychological wellbeing. However, some participants also noted the potential disadvantages and shortcomings associated with the derivation of authenticity. They focused upon the risks of seeking authenticity and, particularly, of authentic self-presentation to others, especially in a potentially hostile social context:

> When I finally admitted I was gay, yes, long term all good but short term really, really bad. There was like a blast of guilt and unhappiness. I was depressed if I'm honest with you. Before that I'd just played along, played the game of "oh maybe I'm straight, maybe I'm bi, or may I'm not" but when you admit it, when I admitted it finally, it affected my feelings about myself. I felt bad. (Sam, gay man)

> I can't explain the feeling. It's weird but when that weight came off my shoulders I actually felt a bit nervous afterwards like something was bothering me and I couldn't put my finger on it but it's the massive seismic shift from being in the closet to finally being yourself and it just feels like a big change and all of a sudden everything changes. It makes you feel a bit distracted, uncomfortable. "Uneasy" is the word. (Peter, bisexual man)

Some interviewees distinguished between the short- and long-term impacts of coming out and specifically referred to the psychological implications of deriving authenticity. For Sam, authenticity at the intrapsychic level, that is, the assimilation-accommodation of his sexuality in identity, had positive long-term implications for identity processes. However, his immediate emotional reaction to assimilating and accommodating his sexuality in identity was that of guilt, which could be attributed to his previous negative feelings in relation to his sexuality. Similarly, Peter reported feeling nervous ("like something was bothering me") when he came out. Internalized homonegativity motivated some individuals to suppress willfully their sexuality and to believe, or rather hope, that they might actually be heterosexual. The psychological transition from sexual identity suppression to assimilation-accommodation can in and of itself represent a threat to continuity. Indeed, Peter described the eventual assimilation-accommodation of his sexuality using the metaphor of a "massive seismic shift."

Continuity could also be challenged in other ways. Some participants anticipated negative reactions to their sexuality upon coming out at the interpersonal level:

> For me, it's like a double-edged sword. Yes, I felt free and open and I could be me but there were the hard bits too because you know you might be accepted a bit less. They may seem OK but there's a lot of work to be done and I couldn't be bothered with it all. I didn't want to have to explain myself to be open, to just be me. (Jill, lesbian woman)

Like Jill, several interviewees feared that there may be negative changes to their relationships with valued others after coming out since there was a risk of rejection: "you know you might be accepted a bit less." Although individuals generally valued their newfound feelings of authenticity, the desire for authenticity competed with the risk of rejection which in turn jeopardized their sense of continuity. Some were uncertain about the link between past, present, and future. Jill expressed concern about the effort that would be required to safeguard valued relationships with others, such as the need to "explain oneself." In short, authenticity—while positive at the intrapsychic level—came at a price at the interpersonal level. There was widespread recognition of the risks associated with seeking authenticity:

> I had to, still have to, constantly remind people that, yes, I'm gay but I'm not like a screaming queen. The whole point for me is being true to myself and when people assume all sorts about me, like "oh, he probably likes partying, fucking everything that moves," all the negative stuff, I have to keep jumping in and saying "I'm different actually." That's the price of coming out too. (Aaron, gay man)

For Aaron, the derivation of authenticity at the intrapsychic level did not necessarily lead to authenticity at the interpersonal level, primarily because of the risk of being stereotyped by others. He clearly sought to differentiate himself from the perceived gay "prototype," which he characterized as "a screaming queen." He feared that his desire for authenticity ("being true to myself") could actually lead to erroneous assumptions from others, especially concerning the values and behaviors perceived to be associated with homosexuality. Therefore, in addition to potential threats to continuity, distinctiveness (in this case, from other gay men) was also imperiled by the desire to be authentic.

Overview

The derivation of identity authenticity was a prominent theme in coming-out individuals' written and interview accounts. Disclosure of their LGB identity to significant others enabled individuals to derive feelings of authenticity, which in turn appeared to enhance other principles of identity, such as self-esteem and self-efficacy. There was a prominent theme of self-discovery and self-certainty in individuals' accounts, suggesting that the derivation of authenticity can also reduce feelings of identity doubt. By coming out, LGB individuals may feel that they can now align their self-presentation with their "true" identity. Yet, some managed their self-presentation in ways that protected other principles of identity while retaining a sense of intrapsychic authenticity. It appeared that an accommodating response from a valued significant other could enhance feelings of identity authenticity, precluding the need to disclose one's LGB identity in all social contexts. In short, it was not deemed necessary to come out to everybody in order to derive feelings of authenticity. LGB people may choose to do so strategically and in contexts deemed to be psychologically "safe." Individuals acknowledged some of the pitfalls of deriving identity authenticity through coming out, such as potential threats to other principles of identity and the possible adverse impact on valued interpersonal relations. Nonetheless, authenticity was pervasively deemed to be a positive outcome of coming out and a motivator for doing so.

References

Apter, M. J. (1983). Negativism and the sense of identity. In G. M. Breakwell (Ed.), *Threatened identities* (pp. 75–90). Wiley.

Birichi, D. K. (2015). *Minority stress and well-being in adult gay men: The mediating role of authenticity.* PhD dissertation, University of Miami, Florida, United States. https://scholarship.miami.edu/esploro/outputs/doctoral/Minority-Stress-and-Well-Being-in-Adult-Gay-Men-The-Mediating-Role-of-Authenticity/991031447633902976

Brownfield, J. M., & Brown, C. (2022). The relations among outness, authenticity, and well-being for bisexual adults. *Psychology of Sexual Orientation and Gender Diversity, 9*(1), 71–80. https://doi.org/10.1037/sgd0000390

Brownfield, J. M., Brown, C., Jeevanba, S. B., & VanMattson, S. B. (2018). More than simply getting bi: An examination of coming out growth for bisexual individuals. *Psychology of Sexual Orientation and Gender Diversity, 5*(2), 220–232. https://doi.org/10.1037/sgd0000282

Cartwright, T., Hulbert-Williams, L., Evans, G., & Hulbert-Williams, N. (2023). Measuring authentic living from internal and external perspectives: A novel measure of self-authenticity. *Social Science & Humanities Open, 8*(1), 100698. https://doi.org/10.1016/j.ssaho.2023.100698

Chen, S., Murphy, D., & Joseph, S. (2024). Dispositional authenticity, internalised homonegativity, and relationship quality in same-gender couples: An actor-partner interdependence moderation model. *Psychology & Sexuality, 15*(1), 127–146. https://doi.org/10.1080/19419899.2023.2231473

DuBois, H. T., & Arena, D. F., Jr. (2023). Bisexual authenticity and job attitudes: The impact of seeing similar others at work. *Journal of Vocational Behavior, 146*, 103918. https://doi.org/10.1016/j.jvb.2023.103918

Fielder, B. (2015). *The negotiation of religious, sexual and gendered identities among lesbian, gay, bisexual and transgender attendees of four church congregations in Australia.* PhD dissertation, University of Tasmania, Australia. https://figshare.utas.edu.au/articles/thesis/Queer_Christianity_-_authentic_selves_the_negotiation_of_religious_sexual_and_gendered_identities_among_lesbian_gay_bisexual_and_transgender_attendees_of_four_church_congregations_in_Australia/23239181?file=40956008

Fletcher, L., & Everly, B. A. (2021). Perceived lesbian, gay, bisexual, and transgender (LGBT) supportive practices and the life satisfaction of LGBT employees: The roles of disclosure, authenticity at work, and identity central-

ity. *Journal of Occupational and Organizational Psychology, 94*(3), 485–508. https://doi.org/10.1111/joop.12336
Franzese, A. (2007). *To thine own self be true? An exploration of authenticity*. PhD Dissertation, Department of Sociology, Duke University, Durham, NC. https://dukespace.lib.duke.edu/items/db982f4f-aa85-4a5a-b614-671fe9fdb0e5
Fredrick, E. G., LaDuke, S. L., & Williams, S. L. (2020). Sexual minority quality of life: The indirect effect of public stigma through self-compassion, authenticity, and internalized stigma. *Stigma and Health, 5*(1), 79–82. https://doi.org/10.1037/sah0000176
Gardner, D. M., & Prasad, J. J. (2022). The consequences of being myself: Understanding authenticity and psychological safety for LGB employees. *Journal of Occupational and Organizational Psychology, 95*(4), 788–797. https://doi.org/10.1111/joop.12399
George, L. (1998). Self and identity in later life: Protecting and enhancing the self. *Journal of Aging and Identity, 3*(3), 133–152. https://doi.org/10.1023/A:1022863632210
Goffman, E. (1963). *Stigma*. Prentice-Hall.
Goffman, E. (1967). *Interaction ritual*. Doubleday.
Guignon, C. (2008). Authenticity. *Philosophy Compass, 3*(2), 277–290. https://doi.org/10.1111/j.1747-9991.2008.00131.x
Hollier, J. (2023). *Religious trauma, queer identities*. Palgrave Macmillan.
Holt, M., & Griffin, C. (2003). Being gay, being straight and being yourself: Local and global reflections on identity, authenticity and the lesbian and gay scene. *European Journal of Cultural Studies, 6*(3), 404–425. https://doi.org/10.1177/13675494030063008
Jaspal, R., & Breakwell, G. M. (Eds.). (2014). *Identity process theory: Identity, social action, and social change*. Cambridge University Press. https://doi.org/10.1017/CBO9781139136983
Jaspal, R., & Breakwell, G. M. (2022). Identity resilience, social support and internalized homonegativity in gay men. *Psychology and Sexuality, 13*(5), 1270–1287. https://doi.org/10.1080/19419899.2021.2016916
Jaspal, R., & Cinnirella, M. (2010). Coping with potentially incompatible identities: Accounts of religious, ethnic and sexual identities from British Pakistani men who identify as Muslim and gay. *British Journal of Social Psychology, 49*(4), 849–870. https://doi.org/10.1348/014466609X485025
Leary, M. R., & Kowalski, R. M. (1990). Impression management: A literature review and two-component model. *Psychological Bulletin, 107*(1), 34–47. https://doi.org/10.1037/0033-2909.107.1.34

Levitt, H. M., Horne, S. G., Herbitter, C., Ippolito, M., Reeves, T., Baggett, L. R., Maxwell, D., Dunnavant, B., & Geiss, M. (2016). Resilience in the face of sexual minority stress: "Choices" between authenticity and self-determination. *Journal of Gay & Lesbian Social Services, 28*(1), 67–91. https://doi.org/10.1080/10538720.2016.1126212

Lovelock, M. (2019). 'My coming out story': Lesbian, gay and bisexual youth identities on YouTube. *International Journal of Cultural Studies, 22*(1), 70–85. https://doi.org/10.1177/1367877917720237

Petrocchi, N., Pistella, J., Salvati, M., Carone, N., Laghi, F., & Baiocco, R. (2020). I embrace my LGB identity: Self-reassurance, social safeness, and the distinctive relevance of authenticity to well-being in Italian lesbians, gay men, and bisexual people. *Sexuality Research & Social Policy, 17*(1), 75–86. https://doi.org/10.1007/s13178-018-0373-6

Rand, J. J., & Paceley, M. S. (2022). Exploring the lived experiences of rural LGBTQ+youth: Navigating identity and authenticity within school and community contexts. *Journal of Gay & Lesbian Social Services, 34*(1), 21–39. https://doi.org/10.1080/10538720.2021.1911902

Riggle, E. D. B., Mohr, J. J., Rostosky, S. S., Fingerhut, A. W., & Balsam, K. F. (2014). A multifactor lesbian, gay, and bisexual positive identity measure (LGB-PIM). *Psychology of Sexual Orientation and Gender Diversity, 1*(4), 398–411. https://doi.org/10.1037/sgd0000057

Riggle, E. D. B., Rostosky, S. S., Black, W. W., & Rosenkrantz, D. E. (2017). Outness, concealment, and authenticity: Associations with LGB individuals' psychological distress and well-being. *Psychology of Sexual Orientation and Gender Diversity, 4*(1), 54–62. https://doi.org/10.1037/sgd0000202

Rostosky, S. S., Cardom, R. D., Hammer, J. H., & Riggle, E. D. B. (2018). LGB positive identity and psychological well-being. *Psychology of Sexual Orientation and Gender Diversity, 5*(4), 482–489. https://doi.org/10.1037/sgd0000298

Roth, D. L., Snyder, C. R., & Pace, L. M. (1986). Dimensions of favorable self-presentation. *Journal of Personality and Social Psychology, 51*(4), 867–874. https://doi.org/10.1037/0022-3514.51.4.867

Russon, J. M., & Schmidt, C. K. (2014). Authenticity and career decision-making self-efficacy in lesbian, gay, and bisexual college students. *Journal of Gay & Lesbian Social Services, 26*(2), 207–221. https://doi.org/10.1080/10538720.2014.891090

Sutton, A. (2020). Living the good life: A meta-analysis of authenticity, well-being and engagement. *Personality and Individual Differences, 153*, 109645. https://doi.org/10.1016/j.paid.2019.109645

Valentine, B. A. (2015). *'Daring to be ourselves': Explorations of authenticity, compassion, and discrimination for lesbian, gay, bisexual, and queer people of color.* PhD dissertation, University of Michigan, United States. https://hdl.handle.net/2027.42/111608

Vannini, P., & Franzese, A. (2008). The authenticity of self: Conceptualization, personal experience, and practice. *Sociology Compass, 2*(5), 1621–1637. https://doi.org/10.1111/j.1751-9020.2008.00151.x

Varga, S. (2014). *Authenticity as an ethical ideal.* Routledge.

Villicana, A. J., Delucio, K., & Biernat, M. (2016). "Coming out" among gay Latino and gay white men: Implications of verbal disclosure for well-being. *Self and Identity, 15*(4), 468–487. https://doi.org/10.1080/15298868.2016.1156568

Williams, K. G. (2023). *Becoming an authentic self: A grounded theory of growth-fostering friendships between gay men.* Unpublished PhD dissertation, Saybrook University, Pasadena, United States. https://www.proquest.com/openview/c5178555b42beff3d04fd78757cedd81/1?pq-origsite=gscholar&cbl=18750&diss=y

6

Enhancing Interpersonal Relationships

Decision-Making Regarding Coming Out

A key concern among people who come out as lesbian, gay, or bisexual (LGB) is the impact that this will have upon their relationships. Some are fearful of the reaction from significant others and therefore decide to conceal their sexuality. There are many factors that underpin the decision to come out as LGB.

In their survey study of 161 LGB people, Legate et al. (2012) found that participants were more likely to come out in contexts that they perceived as autonomy supportive, that is, in contexts in which individuals perceived acceptance and support for their authentic self-expression. In short, people often make assumptions about how their significant others will react to their coming out based upon how supportive they have been previously—often in relation to other matters and identity domains.

Other studies provide further insight into decision-making regarding coming out. Rossi (2010) interviewed 53 gay and lesbian young adults about their experiences of coming out to their parents and found that participants typically came out to their friends before coming out to their parents and that they generally came out to mothers before coming out

R. Jaspal, *The Psychology of Coming Out*,
https://doi.org/10.1007/978-3-032-02599-9_6

to fathers. Interestingly, people generally came out to mothers using direct methods (e.g., sitting them down and telling them) and to fathers using more indirect methods (e.g., asking somebody to tell them on their behalf). These differences may in part be explained by the level of enquiry from particular family members. Indeed, Rossi (2010) found that mothers tended to enquire more about their gay sons' sexuality but less about their lesbian daughters'. Carnelley et al. (2011) conducted a cross-sectional survey study of coming out to parents in a sample of 309 LGB individuals. They found that those participants who perceived their mothers as having been accepting of them in childhood were more likely to come out to their mothers. Those parents who were perceived as more accepting and more encouraging of their child's independence reportedly reacted more positively to their child's coming out. This study too demonstrates the significance of anticipated reactions to decision-making.

Chrisler (2017) proposes a theoretical framework for understanding parental reactions to coming out as LGB that consists of eight stages. One stage basically focuses on the type of reaction from parents which can be neutral, positive, negative, or a combination of some or all of these characteristics. Another is the cognitive and behavioral reaction to coming out which is either active or avoidant. Active cognitive reactions include thinking further about the information given to them by their child and assimilating and accommodating it within their thinking. Active behavioral reactions include seeking further information about their child's sexuality and discussing it further. Avoidant cognitions and behaviors are discussed in Chap. 8. Reactions from significant others appear to have important implications for interpersonal relationships among people who come out.

Reactions to Coming Out

The factors that determine how significant others will react to a loved-one's coming out are complex. The available evidence suggests that individual traits and characteristics, family dynamics, and social and institutional resources all play a role.

McCormack et al. (2014) interviewed 60 gay and bisexual men in the United States and found that the oldest cohort of participants tended to report the most stereotypical and prejudiced reactions to their coming out in contrast to the youngest cohort who reported mainly positive reactions from significant others. They suggest that this reflects a decrease in cultural homonegativity and the changing conceptualization of masculinity itself. van Bergen et al. (2021) analyzed interview excerpts from 155 lesbian, gay, bisexual, transgender, queer, or questioning (LGBTQ) participants using qualitative thematic analysis and found a range of reactions, including suspicion, certainty, and surprise, and a range of appraisals, including silence, invalidation, ambivalence, and validation. Although validating appraisals from parents were most commonly observed in the younger cohorts, invalidating appraisals were actually common across all cohorts. On this basis, the authors challenge the assumption that coming out has become easier for younger people but do note that where the parent-child relationship is characterized by harmony and open communication coming out tends to be experienced positively.

The availability of particular social and institutional resources plays a role in reactions to coming out. Ghosh (2020) argues that a key determinant of parental acceptance of their LGB offspring is access to social resources that can facilitate such acceptance. This can include access to information about LGB identities, support groups, and counselling and family-based therapy. Yet, individual traits and characteristics as well as broader family dynamics appear also to be important factors. In their survey study of 164 LGB young adults in Italy, Baiocco et al. (2015) found that parents' right-wing conservatism, strong religious beliefs, and scoring high on the rigid and enmeshed subscales of the Family Adaptability and Cohesion Evaluation Scale predicted more negative reactions to coming out.

Based upon his interview research with over 150 LGB teenagers, Savin-Williams (2001) puts much emphasis on gender dynamics in relation to coming out, noting, for instance, the differential implications of a gay male coming out to his mother as opposed to his father. He provides a series of recommendations for parents faced with a child's coming out. The support offered by siblings in this process can also be important. Indeed, Haxhe et al. (2018) point to the significant role played by the heterosexual siblings of LGB people who come out, particularly in terms of the socio-emotional support offered to parents and in facilitating feelings of self-acceptance in the coming-out individual.

There is some evidence that a heterosexual parent's own proneness to feelings of shame and guilt is associated with increased likelihood of reacting negatively to their LGB child coming out (Armesto & Weisman, 2001). Furthermore, among fathers in particular, greater masculine honor beliefs (i.e., the belief that it is acceptable to resort to aggressive or violent measures to defend and prove one's masculinity and reputation) are associated with more negative perceptions of their sons who come out as gay as well as a stronger expectation that fathers should reject a son who comes out as gay (Brand & O'Dea, 2022). In their path analysis study of 150 LGB adolescents in Italy, Baiocco et al. (2016) found that lower levels of adaptability and cohesion (which they refer to as poorer family functioning) and strong beliefs in traditional values predicted negative parental reactions to coming out, which in turn was associated with more internalized homonegativity in the adolescents themselves.

Implications for Interpersonal Relationships

Coming out can have multifarious implications for interpersonal relations, such as improving the quality of communication between individuals. However, the relationship between coming out and relational dynamics appears to be moderated by many different factors.

Chandra and Wilkinson (2024) interviewed 15 gay men of South Asian descent about their coming out experiences and found that, for their interviewees at least, coming out appeared to strengthen and enhance their relationships with family members, facilitating friendship, choice, and intimacy with them. More specifically, by coming out, some reported feeling able to repair and even transform their relationships which were often strained due to the silence associated with sexual identity concealment. Communication was greatly enhanced, and there was a sense of openness that they had not previously experienced. An especially noteworthy finding from their study is that, through coming out, family relationships may acquire some intimate qualities that are more akin to chosen friendships. This in turn can strengthen bonds between family members.

Yet, there is also research showing that, in some relational contexts, silence (i.e., not coming out or limiting the extent of one's outness) can be construed as beneficial for some interpersonal relationships. In their analysis of three qualitative datasets on coming out, Nordqvist and Smart (2014) situate coming out in networks of intergenerational relationships and note that hostility in families can shape the coming out process and that silence can sometimes be perceived as maintaining family relationships. They argue that the meanings of LGB identities must be understood in the context of kin relationality.

In families with particular characteristics, such as a strong religious affiliation, the coming out process may need to be managed in particular ways. For instance, in an analysis of the positive aspects of coming out, that is, the sources of family equilibrium following a coming out experience among LGB people raised in conservative Christian families, Drumm et al. (2021) describe the following strategies that can support family equilibrium: parental expression of unconditional love; the passing of time; being in a romantic relationship that can provide interpersonal support; open communication with one's parents; appropriate distance and independence from one's parents; and, in some cases, avoiding sexuality-related topics entirely.

In their study of an ethnically diverse sample of gay and bisexual men's experiences of coming out to their fathers in the United States, Jadwin-Cakmak et al. (2015) found that acceptance came in various different forms and was sometimes characterized by contradictory attitudes toward homosexuality including homonegative and gendered talk. In particular, hegemonic masculinity underpinned many fathers' reactions. In his typographic analysis of 250 coming out stories from LGB people, Manning (2014) identified a series of positive communicative behaviors, such as affirmative statements toward the coming-out individual, laughter and joking, and generally encouraging open communication and conversation. There were also various negative communicative behaviors, whose implications are discussed in Chaps. 8 and 9.

Improvements in Relationships Over Time

It has been shown that even less accepting parents and significant others can be supported to develop more positive and accepting relationships with coming-out loved ones. In an emotional text analysis of semi-structured interviews with 25 parents of coming-out individuals, Carbone et al. (2023) found that, despite the initial challenges in assimilating and accommodating their child's coming out, parents came to develop social networks in which they could share the emotional aspects of being the parent of a LGB child and thereby derive support and offer support to others. This was referred to as family generativity.

LaSala (2000b) describes the potential benefits of therapeutic intervention involving both coming-out LGB individuals and their parents who experience difficulties in accepting their child's sexuality. He argues that both coming-out LGB people and their parents need time and support to learn to relate to one another in non-reactive, non-confrontational ways. This in turn can generate feelings of trust and demonstrate an understanding of the emotional needs of one another. In time, this can facilitate manageable family relationships despite the absence of full parental acceptance of the coming-out person's sexual identity.

In a similar vein, Willoughby and Doty (2010) describe a cognitive behavioral therapy technique specifically for families negotiating the coming out process, whereby parental attributions, beliefs, and expectations regarding their LGB child are explored and challenged. The approach supports the development of specific listening and problem-solving skills so that family members can engage in more adaptive communication. Moreover, based on a literature review, Morrow (2001) proposes a series of guidelines for social work intervention with clients contemplating coming out as LGB to family members. These include *inter alia* understanding identity issues in clients, enabling them to develop a social support system, facilitating practice experiences before actually coming out to family members, and preparing the client for potential upheaval following their coming out experience.

Family dynamics can also be shifted not only to assimilate but also accommodate the coming-out LGB individual in an identity affirmative manner. In their interview study of 8 families, Nascimento and Scorsolini-Comin (2022) noted that, despite initial challenges during the coming out process, over time and in their own way each family was able to build an intelligibility about coming out, which in turn facilitated some level of acceptance. Similarly, Baptist and Allen (2008) argue that, notwithstanding the initial challenges experienced by families during the process of coming out, through the processes of embracing the LGB identity, integrating as a family, building social connections, and experiencing social awakening, families can become accepting of the coming-out LGB person. In an interview study with 10 lesbian women, Coolhart (2006) found that, despite a wide range of parental reactions encountered, participants' relationships with their parents improved significantly over time following the initial coming out event and there was, on the whole, a general sense of acceptance.

The assimilation-accommodation of a coming-out LGB family member is demonstrated in a study of 36 autobiographical accounts of coming out. Gorman-Murray (2008) presents the argument that family homes can become "queered" when an individual comes out as LGB, enabling family members to "resist and subvert heterosexual norms, instead nurturing difference and multifaceted identities" (p. 41). The accounts all suggest that positive reactions to coming out were a precursor to displacing heteronormativity that previously characterized the family home and to unconditional support for the development of LGB identities *within* the family home. Although familial reactions to coming out are not always positive in the first instance, it may be possible to build an infrastructure for acceptance and support in the long term.

Coming out in a religious context can be especially challenging but research provides insight into the facilitators of positive relations over time. In their semi-structured interview study of 23 gay men from Christian and Jewish backgrounds, Etengoff and Daiute (2014) found that religion could also be used adaptively to navigate post-coming out conflicts that emerge in the family. For instance, some significant others used religious mediation, that is, they invoked their faith to mediate conflict that emerged when a loved one came out as LGB.

Consequences of Reactions for Psychological Wellbeing

There is empirical evidence that family (and especially parental) reactions to a LGB person's coming out can have important implications for the coming-out individual's identity and psychological wellbeing. D'Amico et al. (2015) found that parental support of their child's sexual orientation was associated with positive identity and psychological adjustment in the LGB person, while parental struggles with, and attempts to control, the LGB person's sexual orientation were associated with negative identity and psychological adjustment.

In his phenomenological study of 15 Latino gay men's experiences of coming out to their fathers, Gerena (2023) found that, although all interviewees reported favorable reactions to their coming out, they reported struggling with their mental health prior to coming out as they anticipated negative reactions specifically from their fathers. Several interviewees reported consuming alcohol as a means of coping with the psychological stress associated with the prospect of coming out. Legate et al. (2012) studied coming out and psychological wellbeing in a sample 161 LGB people who were more likely to disclose their sexuality in contexts that they deemed to be autonomy supportive rather than controlling.

Valentine et al. (2003) conducted interviews with 20 LGB young adults and described the tension between individuality and collectivity in coming out to significant others within the family. In short, coming out as LGB can have differential implications for the coming-out individual, their parents, their siblings, and others within the broader family structure. One's own self-esteem is contingent not only upon the implications of coming out for oneself but also upon reactions from others.

In their survey study of coming out and post-stress growth in a sample of 102 LGB participants, Solomon et al. (2015) found that negative social reactions from significant others predicted both post-stress growth and depreciation. Cox et al. (2010) similarly found that the more stress-related growth experienced following one's coming out experience, the less internalized homonegativity one reported. It is likely that those who possess resilience and the tools to cope with stress are better positioned to grow from the stress induced by a negative social reaction. Conversely, a positive social reaction following a coming out experience was found to be associated with growth, thereby supporting the development of a healthy LGB identity as well as psychological wellbeing (Solomon et al., 2015).

Lasala (2000a) interviewed 40 coupled gay men regarding the impact of coming out to their parents and in-laws for their own romantic relationship. He found that, despite the challenging aspects of coming out and the initial disapproval almost all interviewees reported, the impact of being out to parents and in-laws was generally deemed to have favorable implications for their relationship. Indeed, even antagonism from parents and in-laws was not perceived as threatening to the relationship since individuals generally maintained a strong sense of independence from their parents and in-laws and maintained intergenerational boundaries.

Written Accounts from Lesbian, Gay, and Bisexual People

In this section, the following three themes arising from the thematic analysis of written accounts from LGB people are reported: (1) continuation of existing relationships; (2) enhancement of existing relationships; and (3) strengthening the family as a whole.

Continuation of Existing Relationships

There was a strong emphasis in participants' narratives about their positive experiences of coming out to someone significant upon the continuation of existing relationships with them. In other words, they valued the fact that nothing appeared to have changed between them as a result of coming out as LGB:

> We still laughed at each other's jokes.

> I told my friend who is male so he would not feel awkward later for not knowing. He did not care. We just partied and hung out like always after.

> We still engaged in the same activities afterwards. We would still go shoot pool, play video games, and hang out with our other friends.

> My relationship with the individual did not change at all after I came out. We were still able to talk and laugh as normal.

In their written accounts, respondents highlighted everyday activities (e.g., laughing together, partying together, and spending time together) that they engaged in and their ability to continue to engage in them without any change after coming out. This was foregrounded as a key aspect of their positive coming out experiences. Continued engagement in these everyday activities with significant others enabled individuals to believe that there remained a continuous thread connecting their past, present, and future. Their relationships were unchanged despite the introduction of novel risky information about their identity, that is, their sexuality. After all, LGB people who decide to come out do not necessarily know for sure how their significant others will react.

In addition to the continuation of everyday activities, the material and emotional support that they received prior to coming out reportedly remained available:

> My mum still supported me with practical help, financial help and continued to communicate in exactly the same way. She still showed she cared and was totally proactive in my life.

> I came out to my mum a few years ago, and it was not a big deal. She's a wonderful woman so she still treats me the same, talks with me and loves me. My relationship with her remained the same.

> I was still able to talk to them as if nothing had changed. They didn't act differently to me. They were there if I needed support and guidance.

Respondents highlighted the continuation of assistance, support, communication, care, guidance, and love. For some, these important material and emotional tenets of their relationship were present before and after coming out. The presence of these tenets following their coming out experience enabled individuals to maintain feelings of continuity in spite of anticipated changes due to coming out. However, it should be noted that some transient change was largely acceptable to individuals provided there were no longer-term changes, as exemplified by the following accounts:

> I remember when I came out to my best straight friend. He was shocked and I think felt really awkward. However one thing that never changed was our friendship. We still do all the same things together and still share the same interests.
>
> Although at the time things changed, it was short lived, our relationship and way of conversation remains the same. We still talk to each other the same amount. We advise each other the same and there is no love lost.
>
> The relationship stayed the same. Although maybe talking about the [subject] for a while the fundamental relationship didn't change.
>
> Essentially, everything stayed the same. Relationships with friends/family/colleagues have been unchanged by coming out. The only exception being my parents, who took a little while to come around, but the relationship essentially was unchanged.

As one of the participants reported, they initially felt "shocked" and "really awkward" when they came out to their best friend but were able to compartmentalize these initial adverse emotional experiences in view of the continuation of their friendship which was clearly of significance to them. The ability to "do all the same things together" and to "still share the same interests" appeared to override these initial negative feelings upon coming out. Another participant acknowledged the need to "talk about the subject for a while," which, for some, can entail having to explain their identity and answer (intrusive) questions, but the experience was deemed to be acceptable because "the fundamental relationship didn't change." This sentiment was expressed more explicitly by another participant who noted that their parent "took a while to come round." This itself can constitute an identity hazard, as this can entail stigmatization and rejection, but on balance this caused no lasting damage to identity since the "relationship essentially was unchanged." In short, some coming-out LGB people appear to differentiate between short- and long-term continuity, clearly tolerating threats to the former.

Identity enhancement stemmed particularly from the contrast between past expectations and the lived experience of coming out to someone who mattered. Several participants noted their feelings of fear and nervousness prior to coming out and the subsequent relief they experienced when their identity was validated by significant others:

> When I was 15 I came out to my gran and I was so scared that she would not accept me being gay but she was the opposite and our relationship stayed the same as it had always been.
>
> I told a friend at university. I was very deeply concerned by this and they said they knew and that was that—it was back to being very close mates.
>
> I was worried when I came out to my best friend. I was afraid our relationship would change. Our friendship has stayed the same through the years.
>
> I told my parents that I was gay, and I was unnecessarily nervous about it. I didn't need to be. Nothing changed in our relationship afterwards.

In some contexts, LGB people are primed to believe that they will face rejection due to the widespread stigmatization of their sexuality in a heteronormative society. They reported relief upon discovering that their relationship had essentially remained the same despite the expectation that there would be negative changes. Continuity clearly underpinned the identity enhancement that they experienced—the relationship was perceived as staying the same but there were also benefits for other principles of identity, most notably, self-esteem:

> Our relationship didn't change and it made me feel validated and good about myself.
>
> We carried on doing the same things and I felt my self-esteem just go up when before it was fragile.
>
> Nothing changed so the shame was replaced by pride.

Some coming-out LGB people do anticipate negative changes subsequent to coming out. However, respondents were pleasantly surprised to learn that there were no changes to their relationships which in turn provided feelings of validation, pride, and general self-esteem. This should be considered against the backdrop of the fear, shame, and anxiety that some LGB people experience before they come out. This can, and often does, take its toll on self-esteem. In addition to the focus upon the continuation of existing relationships, which was especially beneficial for the continuity principle of identity, several respondents highlighted the ways in which coming out enhanced their existing relationships with significant others.

Enhancement of Existing Relationships

Respondents foregrounded the ways in which coming out as LGB had enabled them to think, feel, and act in novel but positive ways in relation to their relationships with significant others.

> When I came out to my parents, the relationship I had with them stayed the same. The support and love I felt was the same as before, if not strengthened by our discussion.

> When coming out to my school friends they were supportive and didn't change the way they treated me. It made our friendships stronger.

Some individuals focused upon the continued derivation of emotional needs, such as support and love, but also indicated this was "strengthened" by coming out to their parents. Similarly, there was reference to the benefits of coming out for the overall quality of their relationships. For instance, one respondent noted that coming out had "made [their] friendships stronger." Thus, the perception that nothing specific changed between them and their significant others when they came out as LGB served to enhance the relationship itself. It is possible that individuals who perceived no change in their relationships upon coming out came to perceive their relationships as resilient and thus valued them more.

Some respondents attributed the enhancement of their existing relationships to their newfound identity authenticity (which was discussed in Chap. 5):

> The amount of support and friendship I received did not change. They were still the same friend to me as before. In fact they were probably a better friend as I didn't have to hide a secret from them.

> I came out and I could be me so it brought us closer and our love for each other grew more.

> After coming out to my parents, my relationship with them improved because I could share more of my life story with them and they are more involved with my life. No aspect has stayed the same with coming out to them.

Some LGB people experience fear and anxiety in relation to coming out and this can lead them to anticipate negative reactions. People may therefore conceal their sexual identity from others although they may not feel entirely comfortable doing so. One participant noted that, because they "didn't have to hide a secret from them," the quality of their friendship with the person to whom they came out improved. Another participant stated that their ability to be authentic ("I could be me") facilitated feelings of closeness and love. Similarly, for some, it was their ability to "share most of [their] life story" with their parents that enhanced their relationship. This reportedly enabled significant others to become "more involved" in their lives. Coming out removed the barriers that previously existed to shield identity from stigma, rejection, and other possible identity hazards. Indeed, for some, this was especially important because coming out confirmed what was already known but never openly discussed:

> I remember the first straight friend I came out to long ago told me she already knew but thanked me for sharing that about myself. We never stopped being friends. Everything remained the same. We visited, spoke on the phone, had lunches.
>
> My mother told me she always knew but never felt comfortable asking me so when I told her it tore down the walls and we have a healthy relationship now. This makes me feel good about myself and it makes up for the past and I feel optimistic about the future.
>
> Came out to my best (female) friend who had a crush on me. She then understood why I never reacted to her feelings in the same way. She then understood me and we became even closer friends. We are closer now, 8 years on, than we have ever been. So I would say our friendship largely remained the same, strong friendship and she stood by me.

When a significant other knows but does not acknowledge one's sexual identity, this can cause a rift in the relationship, limiting the scope of one's conversations and generating anxiety about discussing certain topics lest they cause offence. This is often the result of fear of negative change in the relationship. In a similar vein, one respondent noted the gratitude that their friend had expressed when they came out to them. This essentially removed the barrier that had previously existed—the friend had known but had not raised this with them. This was similarly expressed by another respondent who metaphorically described how coming out as LGB to their mother who "always knew" about their sexuality "tore down the walls" between them. In other words, they became closer and developed a "healthy relationship" as a result. One participant reported that, in disclosing their sexuality to their best friend, they felt that they developed a closer friendship based on greater understanding. Coming out was clearly perceived to be beneficial for the relationship but, as the participant's account suggested, there also appeared to be benefits for the self-esteem and continuity principles of identity. The enhancement of their relationship made them "feel good about [themselves]" (self-esteem) and essentially that the past and future could be aligned favorably (continuity).

For a small number of participants, coming out enhanced their existing relationships in another way. It enabled them to connect with significant others (e.g., siblings, friends) who were also LGB and who, like them, had felt compelled to conceal their sexuality:

> My relationship with my sister, the first person in my family that I came out to after my parents, is virtually unchanged since coming out in 2011. If anything, our relationship has improved because coming out to my sister made her feel comfortable asking me questions and talking through her feelings, which eventually led to her coming out as LGBTQ as well.

> I remember coming out to a female friend only to learn that she was not sure about her sexuality either. Our friendship stayed the same and even became better after that. We are still best friends and I love her so much!

> I was outed and then came out but then this inspired my brother who was married to finally come out and to be free. We are very close and support each other because he has had it hard too.

For these participants, coming out not only enabled them to derive a greater sense of connection with significant others by removing the silence associated with knowing but not acknowledging their LGB identity. Coming out also enabled them to derive a shared sense of experience. In the extracts above, participants noted that their coming out had enabled significant others who were also questioning their sexual identity to share this with them. Their coming out had inspired and empowered others. Participants' accounts showed that this enhanced the existing relationship and enabled them to feel an element of sameness and solidarity. It is also possible that this could enable some to derive personal satisfaction from providing support to their significant others. In short, this shared experience appeared to strengthen bonds between individuals.

Strengthening the Family as a Whole

In reflecting upon the positive aspects of coming out, several participants noted that their coming out experience, though challenging at first, eventually resulted in a strengthening of the family as a whole.

> All the family came together like we hadn't before in the past.
>
> We're a strong and united family now which we weren't before.
>
> Much more cohesion in the family now. We feel more like a family that sticks together.

The written accounts above point to the specific ways in which the family was reportedly strengthened as a result of coming out. This was expressed in terms of the family "coming together," becoming "strong and united," and being characterized by cohesion and solidarity. Crucially, all three respondents attributed this strengthening of the family to their coming out, identifying this as a positive turning-point in their relationship with their significant others. Other respondents elaborated on the challenging relationships they had prior to coming out:

> I judged my parents a lot because I thought they'd hate me but when they didn't I felt bad about myself but good about my family.

> We had a lot of stressful stuff going on because of problems and this [coming out] was a big problem too but we managed to overcome it and just put it to one side. My parents told me that they love me no matter what and my brother did too and so we just came through at the other end.

> Because we got through this despite the religious values of my parents, we all feel like we can get through anything. Like a bullet-proof family.

Respondents had feared rejection from their parents and, in some cases, this was due to homonegativity associated with their religious values. This potentially undermined feelings of self-esteem, but coming out enabled individuals to develop a more positive relationship with their parents and possibly to restore self-esteem. Often, silence surrounding sexuality leads to tense family relations and, thus, by coming out, that is, breaking this silence, some individuals felt that they could develop better relations with them. Some came to recognize the resilience of their family, that is, their ability to bounce back following the initial challenges associated with coming out. Indeed, one participant noted that their family "just came through at the end other end" while another referred metaphorically to their "bullet-proof family." Furthermore, coming out enabled family members to remind each other of their affection and support for one another. Indeed, some indicated that coming out and the subsequent acceptance and inclusion they received from significant others made them feel that they mattered to their loved ones:

> My parents stood up for me when my toxic aunts were slagging me off and this shows that I mean something in the family after all.

> I just sort of felt like a meaningful, important person in my parents' eyes, like I mattered to them.

It was psychologically satisfying for some respondents to discover that their significant others were not only accepting of their sexuality when they came out as LGB but also that they were willing to defend them from homonegativity from others. One participant noted that their parents defended them from homonegative denigration from extended family members, which made them feel that they occupied a meaningful position within the family. Similarly, another stated that, when they came out as LGB and received a positive reaction from their parents, they felt that they "mattered to them." Overall, coming-out individuals' perception that they occupied an important position in their respective families, in spite of their LGB identity, served to dispel previously held fears concerning their future position in the family. This appeared to strengthen the family as a whole.

Interview Accounts from Lesbian, Gay, and Bisexual People

In this section, the following four themes arising from the thematic analysis of the interview accounts are described: (1) relationship continuity; (2) providing a novel channel for open communication; (3) post-conflict trust and intimacy, and post-stress growth; and (4) queering the family home.

Relationship Continuity

As in the written accounts, interviewees also pointed to continuity in significant relationships in the aftermath of coming out as an important determinant of their psychological wellbeing. There was a sense that continuity in the relationship (i.e., things remaining largely the same) was in and of itself a positive outcome of coming out.

> I was most worried about my dad basically but, yes, he was cool with it and we still do the same things and to be fair he doesn't mention it much. It isn't because it's a taboo topic as such. I doubt he'd ask me about my girlfriend if I had one. But he hasn't become cold toward me or overly protective. He is just as he used to be and we have the same relationship as before. (Aaron, gay man)

> Telling your parents is hard because you, well I, felt like it was going to change everything. At worst they'd hate me and at best they'd tolerate me, right? But nothing at all changed when I came out and that just made me feel comfortable about my life as in things can just go on as usual. I had a

> nice childhood and now my adult life was good minus the fear and worry from my childhood. (Jim, bisexual man)

Like Aaron and Jim, several interviewees highlighted their previous fears concerning their parents' reaction to their coming out. Jim entertained the possibility that his father could come to hate him or merely tolerate him. Indeed, in previous research, the psychological pitfalls of "being tolerated" as a LGBT person have been discussed (Cvetkovska et al., 2024). Aaron had considered the possibility that his father could become "cold" or "overly protective" upon learning of his sexual orientation. Yet, in both cases, their parents remained the same, as did their relationship. Indeed, Jim noted that the fact that his relationship with his father did not change when he came out facilitated a greater sense of continuity between his "nice childhood" and current positive life conditions as an openly bisexual man. The only change he highlighted was the current absence of "fear and worry" which had characterized his childhood. By coming out and observing no immediate changes in his valued relationship with his father, Jim no longer felt fear or anxiety. This was echoed by others:

> The thing that gave me a lot of confidence in myself and made me feel "yes, I'm alright" basically that I'm a person of worth, well, it was the fact that our relationship didn't change at all. No weirdness, no extra efforts, no cringeworthy comments about "oh, I'll always love you because you're my son." Just no change as if my sexuality just didn't matter and it shouldn't. That gave me feelings of self-worth. (Bill, gay man)

> The point is nothing changed when I came out and that gave me the power to do it again and again but yes it wasn't always as good and nice as that time but that doesn't really matter because it's the one time that you come out to people who matter to you and that empowers you. (Jill, lesbian woman)

Interviewees often contrasted their actual experience of coming out with their prior expectations regarding it. Bill considered the possibility that his relationship with his father could change or at least that uncomfortable comments or behaviors could ensue. It was implied that exposure to such uncomfortable comments and behaviors could undermine feelings of self-esteem. The fact that he was made to feel that his "sexuality just didn't matter" provided feelings of self-esteem in the face of a possible threat. Furthermore, the stability of his relationship with his father in spite of coming out reassured him that he was "a person of worth."

Like Bill, who noted the positive impact of relationship continuity for his self-confidence, Jill described her coming out experience in relation to her feelings of self-efficacy. Because her relationship with significant others did not change subsequent to coming out to them, she reportedly felt empowered to come out to others. Participants of course reported both positive and negative experiences of coming out to others but, in many cases, just one positive experience of coming out to somebody significant could have a decisive impact on self-efficacy. Crucially, it was the fact that nothing changed in the relationship that enabled individuals to derive feelings of competence and control not only in relation to their current coming out experience but also in relation to future coming out events. They felt psychologically equipped to do so and these feelings of self-efficacy displaced the fear and anxiety many originally reported.

A small number of interviewees expressed mixed feelings toward the relationship continuity that characterized their coming out experience. On the one hand, they acknowledged that this outcome was favorable because it did not entail any changes but, on the other hand, expressed some disappointment that there was little or no reaction to their coming out from their significant others:

> For me it was like a bit of an anti-climax. I expected plates being thrown around the room and got two people who looked at me like it was all just irrelevant, basically nothing happened and nothing changed, but don't get me wrong. I loved that because I didn't feel the way I thought I would, like some weird specimen. I just felt normal. (Michael, gay man)

> Every queer person's worst nightmare, well, mine at least, is to be that stand-out person because of their sexuality. All the assumptions just because you're queer. None of that happened when I came out to my friends because we just carried on being pals and that was what mattered but I was a bit

> like, well, I would have liked a moment to talk about this a bit more, to them, I mean. (Kim, bisexual woman)

> In a way, I kind of wanted them to say something but they did and it was just like "yeah, whatever" and that was fine because my life stayed the same and all but deep down some part of me found that a bit of a disappointment, I'll be honest. (Karen, bisexual woman)

Coming-out LGB people tend to expect some kind of reaction to their coming out but interviewees, on the whole, appreciated the fact that there had been no significant changes to their relationships with significant others. Michael noted that relationship continuity prevented feelings of excessive distinctiveness, which he metaphorically referred to as being made to feel like "some weird specimen" and, similarly, Kim was pleased to have evaded what she described as "every queer person's worst nightmare"—excessive distinctiveness due to her sexuality. Thus, relationship continuity with significant others had positive implications for identity primarily by preventing identity threat. In other words, interviewees did not feel that they stood out because of their sexuality simply because there were no changes in attitude, behavior, or general reaction when they came out.

In spite of the benefits for identity processes, interviewees appeared to lament, to some extent at least, the lack of reaction. Michael had anticipated a negative reaction from his parents and described their reaction "as a bit of an anticlimax," especially in view of his prior expectations. Kim and Karen acknowledged hoping to have the opportunity to discuss their sexuality with their significant others when coming out. In short, they all reported a disappointing end to their coming out given that there appeared to be no significant reaction and certainly no change. They would have valued some acknowledgement of the significance of the coming out event for them. Coming out is of course an important milestone for many LGB people and thus being made to feel "like it was all just irrelevant" and not been given the opportunity to "talk about this a bit more" was an acceptable but suboptimal outcome of their coming out.

Providing a Novel Channel for Open Communication

There was a pervasive view among interviewees that their coming out had provided a novel channel for open communication with their significant others. They often contrasted the silence and trepidation that had previously characterized their relationships with significant others with the open communication that ensued from their coming out:

> I've got to say, coming out has been hard and I don't discuss this with my parents at all but my sister gets me and I can talk to her and that really does mean a lot. I feel like I can open up to her. Before it was denial. Now it's knowing what to say and how to avoid the topic because my parents don't get it but my sister does. We were never close but I can talk to her. She's sort of become a lifeline in that sense. (Deborah, bisexual woman)

Interviewees were of course at different stages of their coming out journey. Some had recently shared their sexuality with significant others while others had done so some time ago. Deborah noted the difficulties associated with her coming out process and that her relationship with her parents still required some attention in order for the family to assimilate and accommodate this novel information about her identity. However, she did point to the positive implications of her coming out for the quality of her relationship with her sister who expressed an understanding of her identity and with whom she developed a more communicative relationship. Coming out can, in some cases, bring together family members who have previously been emotionally distant or even estranged. In Deborah's case, her more communicative relationship with her sister became "a lifeline" especially in the face of the tense relations that ensued from coming out to her parents. This enabled her to exchange confidences with a significant other who made her feel understood. This could at least buffer some of the psychological stress caused by the tensions in her relations with her parents and others. Some interviewees described how their coming out enhanced their relationships:

> There was no substance to our relationship really but this made us talk more and I mean like meaningful deep conversations about stuff that really

> matters rather than the meaningless stuff like "how was your day?" Even those conversations were like censured because if something sexuality-related came up it was like a big no-no. We just opened up more when I came out to them. (Mike, bisexual man)

> We had a superficial relationship, all of us, but now we talk openly about things and therefore we are closer as a family. Talking openly is a big part of any relationship if you think about it and coming out has brought about a better, stronger, more open relationship. (Bill, gay man)

Some individuals evaluated their relationships with significant others prior to coming out as being "superficial" and characterized by "no substance." In some cases, there was a sense of cautiousness in the relationship and certain topics that could lead to discussions about sexuality were deliberately avoided. However, coming out, though challenging at first, did enable some people to develop a more communicative relationship with their parents. Mike noted that his conversations with his parents were no longer superficial but "meaningful deep conversations" about significant matters, rather than "meaningless talk." Similarly, Bill observed that he and his family could not "talk openly about things," which in turn made them "closer as a family." The quality of his relationship with his parents improved significantly after the initial step of coming out and thus transformed the relationship into a stronger one, as noted by others:

> We're still the same family but I do feel like we're more communicative now and we can just say things in a direct way and understand each other more. Things haven't really changed much apart from that and that's all good for the better. (Jamie, bisexual woman)

The perception that coming out had paved the way to greater and more open communication among family members was echoed by other interviewees. Jamie was keen to emphasize relationship continuity in the aftermath of her coming out as a bisexual woman, highlighting greater communication between family members as the only significant *positive* change in their relationship. As a result of coming out, communication between family members was reportedly more direct and underpinned by greater understanding. Indeed, interviewees noted the insidious effects of silence in relation to their sexuality, which could lead to misunderstanding and, in some cases, conflict between family members.

Several interviewees indicated that silence in relation to their sexuality had ramifications for other aspects of their family identity, essentially creating a more general tendency toward silence and superficiality in the relationship. In some cases, this resulted in greater emotional distance between family members as their level of communication and engagement with one another decreased. Coming out reportedly had a more general positive impact on their familial relations:

> I can talk to my parents about a lot more things than I could before if you know what I mean but really the weird thing is that I'm not talking just about my sexuality. There's a lot more we can talk about now without filters. For example, before I would avoid mentioning my cousin getting married or introducing his girlfriend to his parents because I was scared they were going to ask me when I'm introducing my girlfriend to them so I would just avoid the topic altogether. Now there's a lot more transparency and openness. (Chris, gay man)

Chris noted that he and his family just appeared to have relaxed in their relationship which was no longer characterized by cautiousness and trepidation. He reported that they could now talk "without filters" and that the relationship was characterized by "transparency and openness" following his coming out. More generally, interviewees stated that the challenging first step of coming out to their parents amounted to a favorable investment in the future of the relationship. Although the initial phase was often difficult (both prior to coming out and in its immediate aftermath), this first step appeared to open up a line of communication, which, as noted by Chris, positively affected various aspects of identity. He and others simply felt that their relationship improved and that they could move forward and "grow" together as a family.

Post-Conflict Trust and Intimacy, and Post-Stress Growth

As noted throughout this book, coming out experiences are not uniformly positive or negative—they vary. Interviewees reported experiencing negative reactions and even conflict with their significant others upon coming out. These reactions and even their anticipation prior to coming out can result in psychological stress—both for the coming-out LGB individual and their significant others. Interviewees described the development of post-conflict trust and intimacy, and post-stress growth in the family after they came out:

> You know, we had a lot of problems before I came out. We were constantly fighting. There were some innuendos and microaggressions toward me like I'd be going out with a mate and my mum would be giving me that look as if to say "he isn't your mate, is he? You are sleeping with him." That kind of thing. It was like a fight without the actual fight [...] when I told my parents, it was like, yes, the bland response but then something changed and it was like there was honesty now and no hostile kind of behavior from their side. We actually started to feel like a family for the first time. (Aaron, gay man)

Like Aaron, several interviewees described tense familial relations prior to coming out. In some cases, this could be attributed to the knowledge of, but refusal to acknowledge openly, the sexual orientation of the LGB family member. In others, these family tensions could be attributed to the need to conceal and the mistrust that characterized familial relations. In Aaron's case, tensions were particularly high and he and his family were "constantly fighting." Given that Aaron's mother was tacitly aware of, but did not openly discuss, his sexual orientation, she reportedly made "innuendos and microaggressions" toward him, often in relation to his male friends, which in turn heightened tensions in their relationship (see Chap. 9 for a more detailed discussion of microaggressions). All this persisted prior to coming out.

When Aaron did finally come out to his mother, the nature of his relationship with his parents changed for the better—this reportedly paved the way for honesty and decreased hostile behaviors toward one another. Moreover, as implied in his account, they had not previously felt like a family because of the conflict, microaggressions, and innuendos. Coming out enabled them to "feel like a family for the first time." It appeared that the openness, transparency, and clarity that coming out afforded their relationship in turn greatly enhanced it, enabling them all to experience post-conflict trust and intimacy in their relationship.

> I just feel like we trust each other more because I told my parents who I really am and they told me how they really feel about who I am. Basically they always knew but it was hush hush so we didn't talk about it at all. I really think honesty is the best ingredient for a strong family because we were honest and now there's that trust between us. I love my parents. (Peter, bisexual man)

Similarly, Peter described the challenges in his relationship with significant others prior to coming out. Peter noted that his parents had known, but not acknowledged, his bisexuality ("it was hush hush so we didn't talk about it at all"). Coming out reportedly enabled him to reveal his authentic self to his parents and in turn enabled them to comment on it. Overall, the reaction was positive, which in turn paved the way to greater honesty in their relationship. This had previously been lacking precisely because of the silence surrounding his bisexuality. Because of the trust and strength that now characterized his relationship with his parents, he now felt able to love them. This theme was echoed in Julie's account:

> My dad's reaction was pretty bad, more like silence but that felt bad because silence meant shame. My mum reacted badly which made me feel terrible. So all in all, my actual coming out experience was pretty horrific but I'm really glad I did it. I don't regret it for a second actually. I am glad I did it because we're closer as a family now. I think of it as the initial shock of them finding out or like hearing me say it made them react bad but then the guard is down, the barrier is down, and you can just get on with it. We have learned a lot about each other and I'd say we've become quite resilient. (Julie, lesbian woman)

For Julie, the tensions in her relationship with her parents were more significant and deep-rooted. Sometimes the tensions that characterized familial relations culminated in a deeply negative parental reaction to coming out, as exemplified by Julie's account of her coming out experience which she described as "pretty horrific" and attributed primarily to the family's silence in relation to her sexuality. Although these negative parental reactions appeared to affect her psychological wellbeing ("that felt bad"), the longer-term implications of coming out were positive since the family dynamics reportedly improved. Indeed, Julie noted that her ability to discuss openly her sexual orientation with her family removed the "guard" and "barrier" that had previously inhibited their relationship. More generally, her coming out reportedly brought the family closer together since it enabled them to discover more about one another in the absence of silence and other relational barriers. Several interviewees highlighted the positive long-term implications for the family. Julie, for instance, felt that the dramatic change in family dynamics—from conflict to trust and intimacy—demonstrated the family's resilience in the face of challenges. Others also reported the relief they experienced after coming out:

> My parents were just great, they really were. I can't pretend I wasn't scared and I can't pretend it didn't affect my mental health, all that wondering, questioning and fear and all, it took its toll. Telling them was the hardest thing I did and that made me really anxious. But then that with their warmth and love it validated me and we all just grew as a family. (Kim, bisexual woman)

As noted, interviewees often reported anticipating a negative reaction to their coming out, especially from their parents. Kim acknowledged her feelings of fear which in turn affected her overall psychological wellbeing. Coming out can of course be a very difficult, stress-inducing process, as it was for Kim who reported significant uncertainty about the future prior to coming out. The positive reaction that she received from her parents, characterized by warmth, love, and validation, displaced the uncertainty, fear, and anxiety that she had previously experienced. The implications may be positive not only at the individual level (for the coming-out person) but also for the family as a whole: "we all just grew as a family."

In contrast to Kim who focused largely upon her own psychological stress due to anticipated negative reactions from her parents, other interviewees referred to the stress faced by the family as a whole:

> When I came out, especially like in a religious family like mine, it was like a knife cutting through the atmosphere. There was negative energy and vibes around the house. I mean it. Physically I'd go home and I could feel the tension, that there was anger and a lot of tension. That anger and tension translates into anxiety. I know it sounds spiritual but it's true. That anger and tension was making us all feel bad. Mental health in my house when I came out was at a low. But then I broke the ice and we started to talk more and then you could feel that tension going, you know, after the first phase of it all. (Sarah, lesbian woman)

> We were all stressed out because of our own issues. I was stressed because I thought things would never be the same again. They were stressed because I wouldn't give them grandchildren. My sister was stressed because we were stressed but we got over it and there was a silent period and then a growth period for us as a family and now we are over that completely. (Chris, gay man)

Sarah and Chris described the initial psychological stress faced by the entire family when they both came out as LGB. Sarah described this metaphorically in terms of "a knife cutting through the atmosphere" and "negative energy and vibes" and Chris noted simply that they "were all stressed." Sarah elaborated on this psychological stress, noting that the mental health of the entire family was initially challenged when she came out as a lesbian. Several interviewees observed that, in spite of these initial tensions, coming out facilitated another more positive phase in their relationship characterized by growth. In Chris' case, the heightened tensions were followed by "a silent period" and eventually a "growth period for us as a family." For some families, their growth included the effective assimilation-accommodation and positive evaluation of the coming-out person's LGB identity, which is the focus of the next section.

Queering the Family Home

Some interviewees described significant changes that occurred within the family subsequent to their coming out. One longer-term change that occurred in some families concerned the "queering" of the family home, whereby family members "resist and subvert heterosexual norms, instead nurturing difference and multifaceted identities" (Gorman-Murray, 2008, p. 41). This was generally celebrated by participants who observed that their family home had been "queered" after coming out:

> Literally without a doubt the best thing about coming out was that we became a queer family. Obviously I don't mean my dad came out as gay and my mum as a lesbian but we're no longer that heteronormative family that we were before with even me basically feeling ashamed or worried. Now my parents don't just assume all their nephews are straight. They don't make silly comments about LGBTQ+ people. They talk openly and normally about LGBTQ+ people. We're a queer family. (Julie, lesbian woman)

Julie and others described their families as "queer" which meant different things to different people. For Julie, this meant that her family was no longer heteronormative and that sexual diversity (i.e., the possibility that one might actually be LGBTQ) was acknowledged by family members. It is noteworthy that she described the queering of her family as the "best thing about coming out." The queering of her family was manifested in terms of various sexuality-affirmative behaviors among her heterosexual family members. Julie noted, for instance, that her parents no longer assumed that extended family members were heterosexual and that they refrained from making inappropriate remarks about LGBTQ people because of their shift from heteronormativity. Incidentally, Julie noted in passing the negative psychological impact of her family's previous heteronormativity, including feelings of shame and worry. Such changes in attitude and behavior among heterosexual family members signal to the coming-out LGB person that their identity is not only acknowledged but also accepted and valued. This may explain why the queering of the family home was so meaningful to Julie and others who sought feelings of acceptance, inclusion, and validation in the family home.

Similarly, Chris described some of the positive changes that occurred in his family when he came out as gay:

> My mum is so cute so is my dad. Since coming out to them, they ask me naïve questions, it makes me laugh, but I know they mean well. It's not in a judgmental way at all. They ask me stuff so they don't mess things up or put their foot in it, you see what I mean? And then I can see they've remembered it because they'll say or do something hilarious [...] My boyfriend does drag sometimes which they are totally fine with and my mum was like "oh we can go make-up shopping if he wants" and it was cute because she basically just wanted to be considerate. (Chris, gay man)

Chris described the efforts made by his parents to inform themselves about his gay identity which sometimes included posing "naïve questions." However, in contrast to the many interviewees who valued family continuity upon coming out, as reported earlier in this chapter, Chris and others were tolerant of their parents' curiosity about their sexuality as well as changes that subsequently occurred as they learned more about it. They recognized their parents' well-intentioned attempts to understand their sexual identity in order to make them feel more accepted, included, and validated. Chris exemplified this by recounting his mother's offer to accompany his cross-dressing boyfriend to buy makeup. This signaled to Chris his parents' desire to be accepting and accommodating of his sexual identity. These changes were reassuring to coming-out individuals who interpreted them as a queering of the family home.

Some interviewees described their significant others' support for LGB identities in the form of activism. In many cases, this newfound support reflected a significant change, especially as their significant others had initially struggled to assimilate and accommodate the coming out event and its implications:

> I love that my parents and sisters have become LGBT activists basically as in defending the LGBT community really actively and taking a stand on these things because I am a lesbian. It's not just out of respect for me. It's actually because they see this as something that's also relevant to them, to our family, because of me. All this reinforces it's OK to be queer and it gives you that extra bit of self-esteem. (Jen, lesbian woman)

> My mum told me my dad slammed the phone down on his mate because he made a homophobic comment about lesbians. I felt so proud of him. It just shows that this topic is personal for my parents. They're not ashamed of me and they're not afraid of standing up for my rights as a lesbian. It's as though this is part of their identity too, not just mine. (Sally, lesbian woman)

> It was a shock when my brother stood up for me because he had made homophobic comments himself before but it was a full turn once I came out and that did feel good. It made me feel secure. (Aaron, gay man)

All three accounts exemplify the multifarious ways in which significant others come to express their support for their coming-out family member's identity. Jen reported that her parents and sisters actively "defended the LGBT community," while both Sally and Aaron reported that their father and brother, respectively, called out homonegativity from others in defense of their LGB identity. For Aaron, this change was especially significant since his brother had reportedly made homonegative remarks himself before Aaron came out. His coming out precipitated a positive change in his brother's thinking and behavior.

By coming out, individuals made their sexuality relevant not only to their own identities but to those of their significant others. Indeed, Jen stated that her family now viewed sexual diversity as "relevant to them" and Sally noted that it was now "personal" and "part of their identity too." In short, significant others had themselves come to assimilate and accommodate the sexuality of their loved ones into their own family identity. This in turn shaped their attitudes and behaviors in the face of LGB issues and, as clearly demonstrated in the extracts above, homonegativity. It was evident that the queering of the family home in this way provided feelings of self-esteem which, as noted throughout this book, is generally susceptible to threat as LGB anticipate, fear, and experience homonegativity from significant others.

Overview

One of the most positive outcomes of coming out was undoubtedly the enhancement of relationships with significant others. Coming-out individuals generally reported that coming out opened up novel channels for communication where these had previously been absent, since the concealment of their sexual identity had precluded open communication. People now felt able to discuss not only their sexuality but a broader range of topics since they felt closer to their significant others. Indeed, self-disclosure and exchanging confidences do tend to enhance the quality of relationships. In many cases, they derived greater authenticity, as well as self-esteem.

Moreover, coming-out individuals described the favorable impact that their coming out had not only on interpersonal relationships but also on broader social groups they belonged to, most notably their families. People acknowledged that the quality of their relationships with significant others had been suboptimal due to microaggressions and the avoidance of certain topics in view of their sexual identity concealment. Some also acknowledged that initial reactions to their coming out had been challenging. However, in the long term, they generally felt that they and their significant others experienced greater trust, intimacy, and growth subsequent to their coming out. In some cases, families assimilated and accommodated the coming-out individual's sexuality not only by accepting it but also by celebrating, defending, and incorporating it in the family's identity. This provided a further boost to self-esteem in view of the identity hazards to which many reported being exposed due to their (previously concealed) sexuality.

For some coming-out LGB people, the perception that their interpersonal relationships with significant others remained the same in spite of coming out can constitute an important source of continuity amid an unsettling period in which there is uncertainty about the impact that their coming out might have. Coming-out LGB people do not necessarily wish for their sexuality to overshadow other aspects of their identity. This is important especially in view of the multiplicity of identity—one's sexuality is just one aspect of it.

References

Armesto, J. C., & Weisman, A. G. (2001). Attributions and emotional reactions to the identity disclosure ("coming out") of a homosexual child. *Family Process, 40*(2), 145–161. https://doi.org/10.1111/j.1545-5300.2001.4020100145.x

Baiocco, R., Fontanesi, L., Santamaria, F., Ioverno, S., Baumgartner, E., & Laghi, F. (2016). Coming out during adolescence: Perceived parents' reactions and internalized sexual stigma. *Journal of Health Psychology, 21*(8), 1809–1813. https://doi.org/10.1177/1359105314564019

Baiocco, R., Fontanesi, L., Santamaria, F., Ioverno, S., Marasco, B., Baumgartner, E., Willoughby, B. L. B., & Laghi, F. (2015). Negative parental responses to coming out and family functioning in a sample of lesbian and gay young adults. *Journal of Child and Family Studies, 24*(5), 1490–1500. https://doi.org/10.1007/s10826-014-9954-z

Baptist, J. A., & Allen, K. R. (2008). A family's coming out process: Systemic change and multiple realities. *Contemporary Family Therapy: An International Journal, 30*(2), 92–110. https://doi.org/10.1007/s10591-008-9057-3

Brand, O. R., & O'Dea, C. J. (2022). Less of a man? Masculine honor beliefs influence perceptions of hypothetical sons (and their fathers) coming out as gay. *Personality and Individual Differences, 186*(Part A), 111361. https://doi.org/10.1016/j.paid.2021.111361

Carbone, A., Pistella, J., Gennaro, A., Petrocchi, C., & Baiocco, R. (2023). Parental experiences of coming out: From "un-doing family bonds" to "family generativity". *Journal of Homosexuality, 70*(10), 2135–2157. https://doi.org/10.1080/00918369.2022.2048334

Carnelley, K. B., Hepper, E. G., Hicks, C., & Turner, W. (2011). Perceived parental reactions to coming out, attachment, and romantic relationship views. *Attachment & Human Development, 13*(3), 217–236. https://doi.org/10.1080/14616734.2011.563828

Chandra, S., & Wilkinson, J. (2024). Making friends with the family: A fresh look at coming out. *Journal of Sociology, 60*(2), 311–328. https://doi.org/10.1177/14407833221146785

Chrisler, A. J. (2017). Understanding parent reactions to coming out as lesbian, gay, or bisexual: A theoretical framework. *Journal of Family Theory & Review, 9*(2), 165–181. https://doi.org/10.1111/jftr.12194

Coolhart, D. A. (2006). *Sexual minority women: Exploring familial relationship development after coming out at home*. PhD dissertation, Syracuse University. https://surface.syr.edu/mft_etd/24/

Cox, N., Dewaele, A., van Houtte, M., & Vincke, J. (2010). Stress-related growth, coming out, and internalized homonegativity in lesbian, gay, and bisexual youth. An examination of stress-related growth within the minority stress model. *Journal of Homosexuality, 58*(1), 117–137. https://doi.org/10.1080/00918369.2011.533631

Cvetkovska, S., Jaspal, R., Verkuyten, M., & Adelson, L. (2024). Coping with being tolerated: Trans experiences. *Psychology of Sexual Orientation and Gender Diversity, 11*(1), 31–41. https://doi.org/10.1037/sgd0000580

D'Amico, E., Julien, D., Tremblay, N., & Chartrand, E. (2015). Gay, lesbian, and bisexual youths coming out to their Parents: Parental reactions and youths' outcomes. *Journal of GLBT Family Studies, 11*(5), 411–437. https://doi.org/10.1080/1550428X.2014.981627

Drumm, R. D., Sedlacek, D. A., VanderWaal, C. J., Trecartin, S. M., & Carbonell, N. J. (2021). "Life is Getting Better": Understanding stabilizing factors in conservative Christian families post-coming out. *Journal of GLBT Family Studies, 17*(2), 135–149. https://doi.org/10.1080/1550428X.2020.1800544

Etengoff, C., & Daiute, C. (2014). Family members' uses of religion in post–coming-out conflicts with their gay relative. *Psychology of Religion and Spirituality, 6*(1), 33–43. https://doi.org/10.1037/a0035198

Gerena, C. E. (2023). The coming out experience of Latino gay men. *Families in Society, 104*(2), 101–110. https://doi.org/10.1177/10443894211039836

Ghosh, A. (2020). After coming out: Parental acceptance of young lesbian and gay people. *Sociology Compass, 14*(1), e12740. https://doi.org/10.1111/soc4.12740

Gorman-Murray, A. (2008). Queering the family home: Narratives from gay, lesbian and bisexual youth coming out in supportive family homes in Australia. *Gender, Place and Culture, 15*(1), 31–44. https://doi.org/10.1080/09663690701817501

Haxhe, S., Cerezo, A., Bergfeld, J., & Walloch, J. C. (2018). Siblings and the coming-out process: A comparative case study. *Journal of Homosexuality, 65*(4), 407–426. https://doi.org/10.1080/00918369.2017.1321349

Jadwin-Cakmak, L. A., Pingel, E. S., Harper, G. W., & Bauermeister, J. A. (2015). Coming out to dad: Young gay and bisexual men's experiences disclosing same-sex attraction to their fathers. *American Journal of Men's Health, 9*(4), 274–288. https://doi.org/10.1177/1557988314539993

Lasala, M. C. (2000a). Gay male couples: The importance of coming out and being out to parents. *Journal of Homosexuality, 39*(2), 47–71. https://doi.org/10.1300/J082v39n02_03

LaSala, M. C. (2000b). Lesbians, gay men, and their parents: Family therapy for the coming-out crisis. *Family Process, 39*(1), 67–81. https://doi.org/10.1111/j.1545-5300.2000.39108.x

Legate, N., Ryan, R. M., & Weinstein, N. (2012). Is coming out always a "good thing"? Exploring the relations of autonomy support, outness, and wellness for lesbian, gay, and bisexual individuals. *Social Psychological and Personality Science, 3*(2), 145–152. https://doi.org/10.1177/1948550611411929

Manning, J. (2014). Positive and negative communicative behaviors in coming-out conversations. *Journal of Homosexuality, 62*(1), 67–97. https://doi.org/10.1080/00918369.2014.957127

McCormack, M., Anderson, E., & Adams, A. (2014). Cohort effect on the coming out experiences of bisexual men. *Sociology, 48*(6), 1207–1223. https://doi.org/10.1177/0038038513518851

Morrow, D. F. (2001). Coming out to families: Guidelines for intervention with gay and lesbian clients. *Journal of Family Social Work, 5*(2), 53–66. https://doi.org/10.1300/J039v05n02_05

Nascimento, G. C. M., & Scorsolini-Comin, F. (2022). Coming out in families of gay and lesbian people. In N. A. de Morais, F. Scorsolini-Comin, & E. Cerqueira-Santos (Eds.), *Parenting and couple relationships among LGBTQ+ people in diverse contexts* (pp. 41–56). Springer.

Nordqvist, P., & Smart, C. (2014). Troubling the family: Coming out as lesbian and gay. *Family, Relations and Societies, 3*(1), 97–112. https://doi.org/10.1332/204674313X667380

Rossi, N. E. (2010). "Coming out" stories of gay and lesbian young adults. *Journal of Homosexuality, 57*(9), 1174–1191. https://doi.org/10.1080/00918369.2010.508330

Savin-Williams, R. C. (2001). *Mom, dad. I'm gay. How families negotiate coming out.* American Psychological Association. https://doi.org/10.1037/10437-000

Solomon, D., McAbee, J., Åsberg, K., & McGee, A. (2015). Coming out and the potential for growth in sexual minorities: The role of social reactions and internalized homonegativity. *Journal of Homosexuality, 62*(11), 1512–1538. https://doi.org/10.1080/00918369.2015.1073032

Valentine, G., Skelton, T., & Butler, R. (2003). Coming out and outcomes: Negotiating lesbian and gay identities with, and in, the family. *Environment and Planning D, 21*(4), 479–499. https://doi.org/10.1068/d277t

van Bergen, D. D., Wilson, B. D. M., Russell, S. T., Gordon, A. G., & Rothblum, E. D. (2021). Parental responses to coming out by lesbian, gay, bisexual, queer, pansexual, or two-spirited people across three age cohorts. *Journal of Marriage and Family, 83*(4), 1116–1133. https://doi.org/10.1111/jomf.12731

Willoughby, B. L. B., & Doty, N. D. (2010). Brief cognitive behavioral family therapy following a child's coming out: A case report. *Cognitive and Behavioral Practice, 17*(1), 37–44. https://doi.org/10.1016/j.cbpra.2009.04.006

7

Rejection, Emotional Distance, and Ambiguous Loss

Manifestations of Rejection

For decades, empirical research has shown that lesbian, gay, and bisexual (LGB) people fear rejection, discrimination, and harassment from family members, which in turn can discourage them from coming out (e.g., Ben-Ari, 1995a; Cramer & Roach, 1998). Rejection occurs when one is not accepted and included in a social group or dyad. It can also be thought of in terms of the withdrawal of support. Support itself has many distinct forms which can be financial, emotional, romantic, and social (Cafferty, 2017). Studies indicate that rejection is qualitatively different from just negative responses to one's sexuality (Ben-Ari, 1995b; Carastathis et al., 2017; Samarova et al., 2014; Smith et al., 2020). After all, significant others may be disapproving of the coming-out individual's sexuality but make it clear to them that they remain accepted, included, and loved.

In an interview study of 60 bisexual men and women, McLean (2007) notes the particular challenges faced by individuals in relation to coming out and especially the anticipation that their bisexual identities will not be understood or accepted by significant others. This can lead some people to conceal their bisexual identity and to feign heterosexuality, which

R. Jaspal, *The Psychology of Coming Out*,
https://doi.org/10.1007/978-3-032-02599-9_7

itself can constitute a source of shame. McLean critiques the social imperative to come out in order to live authentically since this often overlooks the social and psychological pressures faced by LGB people.

In view of the flawed notion that homosexuality can be attributed to poor parenting, coupled with general societal stigma toward homosexuality, it is perhaps unsurprising that some parents react negatively to their child's coming out, sometimes using the threat of exclusion, rejection, or estrangement as a means of attempting to change their child's sexuality (LaSala, 2000). Hostility from parents may reflect their own beliefs and values in relation to their child's sexuality as well as their desire to change it (D'Amico et al., 2015). Parents may believe that they have failed in their duty and react defensively by rejecting their coming-out child (Jaspal, 2020).

Pollitt et al. (2023) note the complexity of family environment in the context of coming out as LGB, highlighting that the family environment of many coming-out LGB people is characterized simultaneously by positive and negative behaviors from family members. They therefore call for research into both accepting and undermining behaviors from family members to understand the family environment more fully. In a typographic analysis of 258 coming out narratives from 130 LGB people, Manning (2015) found that negative experiences of coming out were characterized by shaming and aggressive statements and, in some cases, religious talk, all of which were interpreted by the coming-out individual as non-acceptance and possibly rejection of their sexual identity. In two waves of interviews with 15 lesbian, gay, bisexual, and transgender (LGBT) people, DeChants et al. (2022) found evidence of many forms of perceived parental rejection, including increased conflict, silence and avoidance, and control and isolation. Their qualitative data indicated a series of negative psychological and emotional reactions to such rejection.

In their interview study of 21 gay men and lesbian women in Australia, Carastathis et al. (2017) found that family rejection could be either overt or subtle. Yet, both reinforced the perception that the coming out individual's sexual identity was flawed. In some cases, there was continued rejection after the initial coming out experience with the coming-out individual's sexual identity essentially remaining a barrier in the relationship. The authors also describe the concept of conditional love, whereby family acceptance, love, and affection are felt to be available to the LGB individual only on the condition that they change their sexuality and adopt heterosexuality. The authors note the adverse effects for identity and psychological wellbeing and outline a series of strategies that may be used by coming-out LGB people in order to cope, such as strategic outness (i.e., coming out selectively) and sexual identity concealment.

Sense of Loss

The prospect and act of coming out can induce feelings of loss. In particular, coming-out individuals may believe that they will lose valued relationships. Thompson (1996) describes a five-stage model of loss that can accompany coming out as LGB. Stages include acknowledgement of the loss of heterosexual identity upon coming out, understanding the specific elements of the loss (e.g., loss of relationships) and seeking ways of adjusting to it, and the assimilation-accommodation of novel identity elements as a LGB person. Loss and indeed emotional distance can arise from the divergent expectations that LGB people and their significant others have regarding one another prior to the coming out event (Jhang, 2018). While significant others (especially parents) may have heteronormative expectations, coming-out LGB people often expect acceptance and inclusion from their significant others. In their feminist grounded theory study, Rickards and Wuest (2006) found that one of the challenges that LGB people who come out at mid-life may experience is the initial loss of credibility (from valued others) in relation to their identity, which many nonetheless strive to regain.

In their interview study of 12 men who used Facebook to come out as gay, Chester et al. (2016) found that several interviewees had previously experienced homonegativity, especially from significant others, prior to coming out online. This in part led them to anticipate negative reactions from them, including possible loss of the relationship itself, when they decided to come out online. A unique type of loss experienced on social media was the act of being "unfriended" by others, sometimes without explanation, following one's sexual identity disclosure. This may constitute an ambiguous loss because no explicit discussion has taken place—the relationship is simply discontinued in the online context. The emotional distance and sense of loss associated with coming out as LGB people have also been described in terms of disenfranchised grief (Meris, 2023; Wheat & Thacker, 2019).

In an analysis of qualitative material from a study of LGB people using tenets of ambiguous loss theory, Dziengel (2015) argues that LGB people who come out may experience a sense of loss which is ambiguous given that the "lost" family member may, in some cases, remain physically present but become psychologically absent and, in others, become physically absent but remain psychologically present. Family members may become emotionally distant and change the way in which they relate to the coming-out individual. They may be perceived by the LGB person as being "cold" toward them. They may subtly exclude the coming-out person from the family by "accidentally" forgetting to invite them to family functions or making requests that amount to exclusion, such as asking that the LGB person's partner not be included in family events or photographs.

Ambiguous loss may be difficult to identify and may not be immediately recognized by others but, as it amounts to unresolved grief, is poignant for the coming-out LGB person who experiences it. The experience of ambiguous loss can be psychologically stressful and may lead the coming-out LGB person to question their role and position within the family or social group, their sense of belonging within it, as well as their overall self-esteem. Dziengel (2015) noted in her study that some participants observed that their significant others no longer related to them in quite the same way as they did before, representing an ambiguous loss. In some cases, this was signaled by a change in the nature or depth of communication that they had enjoyed prior to the coming out event. In short, significant others were physically but not psychologically present, as per ambiguous loss theory. Although some reached resolution over time, a sizeable number of respondents noted that their significant others were now "more" and "mostly" accepting, suggesting that there was not complete resolution and closure.

Psychological Consequences of Rejection, Emotional Distance, and Loss

Empirical research shows that the effects for psychological wellbeing of rejection, emotional distance, and loss are generally negative. Drawing upon case studies of people coming out as LGB, Sand (2015) observes that "[t]he possibility of being judged unacceptable elicits real and imagined fears of estrangement and of the loss of relational connectedness" (p. 262). It is important to acknowledge that fear of loss of valued interpersonal relationships can undermine mental health outcomes, potentially precipitating distress, anxiety, and depression. Furthermore, she notes that LGB people may experience guilt when they receive a reaction that suggests that they have not met the (heterosexist) expectations of significant others. The identity hazard of rejection (however subtle) can in turn become internalized, resulting in self-hatred.

Although the coming out process often culminates in acceptance of the LGB individual and can, as the previous chapter describes, strengthen relationships, the undoing of family bonds is a common step within this process, which can be distressing for the coming-out LGB person as well as their family members (Carbone et al., 2023; Ghosh, 2020; Jaspal, 2020). Rejection due to one's sexual identity is associated with increased loneliness (Giano et al., 2022). It has also been shown that parental rejection is associated with the development of personality psychopathology, such as negative affect, detachment, and identity impairment (Davis & Anderson, 2021). It has similarly been found that perceived alienation from significant others following coming out is positively associated with current attachment insecurity (Rejiester, 2014).

There is now considerable empirical evidence concerning the relation between exposure to stigma (and indeed other identity hazards) and poor health and wellbeing outcomes (Bird et al., 2017; Ryan et al., 2009; Valdiserri et al., 2019). In this chapter, identity hazards emanating from significant others (most notably one's family) are examined, focusing on the specific psychological burden of emotional distance from and perceived loss of significant others in one's life. Parental support has been found to be associated with lower suicidal ideation among LGB youth

(Hatchel et al., 2019). Parental rejection has been found to be associated with the development of sexual identity struggles while family support facilitates the development of a positive sexual identity (Taylor & Neppl, 2023). Conversely, in a meta-analysis (de Lange et al., 2022), negative family treatment was found to be positively associated with suicidal ideation. Using path analysis, Willoughby et al. (2010) found that family rejection experiences were associated with psychological distress via negative LGB identity, suggesting that when family rejection experiences precipitate internalized homonegativity (i.e., negative LGB identity) LGB people are more likely to experience psychological distress. Moreover, rejection from one's family of origin has been found to be associated with suicidal ideation via depressive symptoms (VanBergen & Love, 2022).

In their survey of 198 people, Hill and Pettit (2012) found that the indirect relationship between being LGB and suicidal ideation via perceived burdensomeness (i.e., the perception that one is a burden on others) was conditional on the perceived level of rejection from others. In other words, those who anticipated or perceived rejection from significant others were more likely to feel like a burden on others which in turn was associated with increased suicidal ideation. In their multiple regression analyses using the Parental Acceptance and Rejection of Sexual Orientation Scale, Kibrik et al. (2019) found that perceived maternal rejection was lower than perceived paternal rejection among gay and bisexual sons and that, for LGB people more generally, acceptance and rejection predicted psychological wellbeing. Indeed, the extent of family support in relation to one's sexuality has been found to be predictive of several wellbeing outcomes, including internalized homonegativity and binegativity, depression, and lower life satisfaction (Sheets & Mohr, 2009).

In their survey study of 309 LGB people, Enderwitz et al. (2024) found that perceived parental rejection was associated with poor mental health outcomes (i.e., depression, anxiety, and stress) and negatively correlated with self-acceptance. Furthermore, they found that self-acceptance moderated the relationship between perceived parental rejection and current psychological distress, suggesting that the relationship between perceived parental rejection and distress is stronger for those LGB people who develop low self-acceptance compared to those who do not.

In their survey study of 108 LGB people, Ryan et al. (2015) found that a negative reaction from a significant other was associated with both higher depression and lower self-esteem and that this relationship was mediated by autonomy need satisfaction, that is, the perception that one can truly be oneself around others. It is noteworthy that reporting a positive reaction from a significant other was not associated with the wellbeing measures. These results suggest that a negative reaction from a significant other may signal to the coming-out individual that they cannot act authentically around them, which in turn may undermine their psychological wellbeing. They also highlight the potentially lasting effects of a negative coming out reaction.

In their survey study of 8774 LGBT adolescents, Meanley et al. (2021) found that familial warmth (i.e., perceived closeness and the expression of love and affection) and self-esteem were positively correlated, while familial rejection and self-esteem were negatively correlated. Furthermore, in their study, family rejection moderated the relationship between familial warmth and self-esteem, essentially attenuating the relationship, suggesting that familial warmth and family rejection are not mutually exclusive experiences among LGB people.

Some studies comparing various wellbeing outcomes between those who do and those who do not come out have found that LGB people who are out generally report more feelings of acceptance and less rejection from parents and less engagement in maladaptive behaviors, such as substance misuse (e.g., D'Amico & Julien, 2012). In a study of 427 LGB people (Macbeth et al., 2022), it was found that the relationship between perceived parental religiosity and poor mental health/substance misuse was mediated by perceived familial stigma of one's sexuality. It may be that religiosity heightens the likelihood of stigmatizing LGB people which in turn is associated with poorer mental health outcomes and likelihood of misusing substances to cope. It must be noted that the mediator of familial stigma is important because it is possible for religion to be used favorably in order to assimilate and accommodate the LGB identity of the coming-out individual (Etengoff & Daiute, 2014).

Challenges associated with coming out can be more significant for people from some ethnic and cultural backgrounds. Most of the interviewees who participated in a study of queer Latino college men's coming out experiences (Eaton & Rios, 2017) reported encountering negative reactions to their coming out, including the loss of valued relationships. In a study of an ethnically diverse sample of LGB people (Dorri et al., 2024), it was found that a series of adverse communication styles emerged in families in relation to coming out, including silence and ignoring, both indicative of emotional distance and (at least partial) loss of relationship. There were particular challenges reported by Black and Hispanic interviewees surrounding the implications of coming out for the family's reputation (see also Jaspal, 2020). Jaspal and colleagues (Jaspal & Cinnirella, 2010, 2012; Jaspal & Siraj, 2011) describe the significant psychological challenges that British Muslim gay men face when contemplating coming out to significant others due to perceived incompatibilities between their sexuality and religion. Similar empirical patterns are also observed in British South Asian gay men from other religious backgrounds (Jaspal, 2012).

Written Accounts from Lesbian, Gay, and Bisexual People

In this section, the following three themes arising from the thematic analysis of written accounts from LGB people are reported: (1) tension and loss in relationships; (2) emotional distance; and (3) religion and culture as lenses for interpreting coming out.

Tension and Loss in Relationships

Some respondents described the tension that came to characterize their relationships with others when they came out to them, which, in some cases, culminated in a sense of loss:

> It's made the relationship a bit more tense with my parents.

> A friend at university over 20 years ago (who also happened to be an attractive, well-built heterosexual male). Although there were no overt signs that he was acting negatively, he did seem awkward. The friendship broke down shortly afterwards.

> When I came out to my best mate several years ago I expected him to be understanding about it, but he was not and did not contact me or text/call for several months.

These accounts exemplify the negative impact of coming out for close interpersonal relationships. One individual described his relationship with his parents as "tense." Another indicated that his heterosexual male friend seemed "awkward" when he came out to him, subsequently leading to the breakdown of their friendship. Similarly, another respondent's friend was, contrary to expectations, not understanding toward them and contact was subsequently lost. While reactions were qualitatively different, they all foregrounded the relational tension that was experienced by coming-out individuals.

The decline and, sometimes, rupture in coming-out individuals' relationships could be attributed to several factors, including the assumption that they might be sexually attracted to the person to whom they were disclosing their sexuality:

> A few years ago, I used to have a really good friend, but I told him I was a gay, and then he started acting weirdly, until we lost all forms of contact. I think he probably thought I was into him. That's the only bad experience I've had with a close person.

> One of my close friends who is a male now does not hang out with me much anymore as a result of me coming out to him. He thinks that I might be into him even though that is not the case at all.

> My cousin started making uncomfortable comments such as "Just make sure you remember I'm not gay" to imply that I might be looking at him in that way. It made me feel really horrible actually.

Sexuality is of course just one element of the coming-out individual's identity. In these cases, this identity element appeared to be foregrounded by others and the friendship was viewed primarily through this lens, thereby engendering concerns that one might be propositioned. Bearing in mind the observation in the previous chapter that individuals valued the continuation of previous activities with their significant others, it is easy to see why this emotional distance followed by complete loss would be challenging for the individual's identity. This could create tensions in their relations with significant others, overshadowing the relationship and causing them to overthink. Respondents referred to the sense of loss that ensued from these tensions:

> When I came out to my sister, there was an unnecessary tension from then on as if there were now boundaries and some off-limits topics so that was a negative change that happened.
>
> We kept our relationship but there was something that was lost when I came out. My mother and I had this weird tension in our relationship.
>
> My parents and I just grew apart after that. There was a kind of distance between us that made me miss the complete relationship we had before all that happened.

Although there was not necessarily overt discrimination, coming-out individuals interpreted the "unnecessary tension," "boundaries," and "distance" as evidence that their sexual identity was not acceptable. For some, this represented negative change in their relationships with valued others—they longed for the intimacy that had previously characterized these relationships. Individuals described the tension in the atmosphere and decreased sense of belonging that they derived after coming out as LGB:

> You could almost cut the tension with a knife and this was the most negative bit about coming out for me.
>
> There was a negative energy after I came out. Not blatant discrimination but home was not really a place I could call home anymore because of those negative vibes. I used to dread coming home after that.

Negative reactions to coming out were not always overt but they were nevertheless perceptible. Respondents referred to the "tension," "negative energy," and "negative vibes" that they perceived and, in some cases, felt that they were no longer accepted and included in spaces that they had previously considered to be safe, such as the family home. This could be attributed to the negative changes in their relationships with significant others, whose negative consequences for identity and psychological well-being were palpable:

> My best friend grew apart and we lost our friendship because he changed as soon as I told him I'm gay. First, there was distance and then our friendship just ran its course. That made me question a lot about life. You can't predict anything, including friendships.

> My brother and I were close. I came out to him. We were on eggshells. Made me feel really sad actually.

These extracts illustrate the psychological effects of the emotional distance and loss that coming-out individuals experienced. Several individuals described feelings of sadness due to the perceived loss of their relationship with significant others. Some clearly found the distance that followed their coming out experience to be unexpected and thus threatening for their sense of continuity. One participant described his sense that he could no longer predict future events or the continuity of his friendships, which could make individuals feel sensitive and anxious about future rejection associated with coming out. It is easy to see how this could discourage some LGB people from coming out to others in the future.

Emotional Distance

Several respondents described how open acknowledgement of information that in some cases was already known by others caused greater emotional distance. This emotional distance arose because coming out was perceived by significant others as a threat to family cohesion and identity:

> My father told me that he had assumed I was gay, but didn't want me to tell him. He was from then even more distant to me than before.

> When I came out to my parents, they experienced a sense of grief at not having grandchildren. Although I could understand their upset to an extent, it suggested a level of ignorance about homosexual relationships and different family structures. This subtly changed my opinion of my parents because of their unexpected reaction.

> This person that I came out to stopped seeing my future as promising and fulfilling. They see me now that I am some sort of failure or anchor to the family dragging its future into one of incontinuity though there has been some understanding and love. I've talked to them about my immorality and disobedience to God's commands quite frequently, so I would say that's certainly a negative that I am looked at as some disgrace to the family and to God.

All three participants indicated in one way or another that their coming out was construed as a threat to the family. It is noteworthy that all these experiences were said to result in some form of emotional distance. One respondent indicated that his father had known but preferred not to acknowledge his sexuality—having to acknowledge his son's sexual identity made him "more distant" toward his son. For another respondent, the threat to the family was manifested in terms of their parents' "ignorance about homosexual relationships and different family structures." Their parents reportedly assumed that they would never be grandparents which led them to experience "a sense of grief," further stigmatizing the individual's sexual identity instead of providing support. This experience should be contrasted with the psychological benefits—especially that of support acquisition—described in the previous chapter. One participant noted that the family member they came out to came to view them as "some sort of failure or anchor to the family" and their future as no longer "promising and fulfilling" because of their sexuality. Though they acknowledged "some understanding and love," coming out was essentially construed as a threat.

> My sister was really cold after I told her about my sexuality. I felt like I failed my whole family.

> When I came out to my parents, they just said nothing but I did feel like I wasn't wanted there anymore. They seemed to be waiting for me to tell them I was going and that felt bad.

> My best friend at the time stopped being my best friend because we stopped having the conversations we used to have although we did not have any fight.

Emotional distance may occur because the coming-out individual is perceived as a threat of some kind to the family. One participant reported that he himself felt that he had "failed" his family by coming out as gay. This view was reinforced by his sister's subsequent behavior toward him—she was reportedly "really cold," indicating that she became emotionally distant from him. Similarly, another respondent noted that, although nothing explicit was said about his sexuality after he came out to his parents, he felt unwanted and believed that his parents wanted him to leave home. One of the most insidious aspects of this type of behavior was the uncertainty that individuals experienced. They were not unequivocally rejected but perceived an emotional distance which they could attribute only to their decision to come out. Indeed, one participant noted that their best friend grew distant from them, indicated by the abrupt end to the close contact that they previously had, when they came out to them.

The emotional distance that individuals perceived from significant others subsequent to coming out had broader ramifications for their lives since they had previously been reliant upon these individuals for support:

> When I told my mum, she disconnected from me on an emotional level. If I was sad, she didn't seem to see it like she did before. She couldn't comfort me about everyday problems because she didn't agree with my lifestyle.
>
> My cousin and I became emotionally distant. We had been close until that point but I could tell she judged me and so we just drifted apart.
>
> Before my parents and I could talk about most topics but not my sexuality. When I came out to them, this immediately created a barrier that meant I could not talk about most things. We stopped talking and stopped understanding each other. It was an emotional break-up in a way.

One respondent recounted the emotional disconnection from their mother after coming out, which meant that she ceased to be a source of support for them. The notion that their mother disagreed with their sexual identity was perceived as a barrier to support. Similarly, another respondent felt judged by their cousin with whom they had previously enjoyed a close relationship. They became "emotionally distant" after the coming out event. Although, for some LGB people, coming out can strengthen and enhance interpersonal relations, there are clearly cases of estrangement, as highlighted in the accounts above. One respondent powerfully communicated this by using the metaphor of an "emotional break-up" with their parents after they came out to them. Although the topic of his sexuality had always been off-limits, they had otherwise enjoyed a fairly close relationship that permitted the discussion of many other topics. They reported that the relationship became constrained after coming out which "immediately created a barrier." They ceased to communicate and understand one another as they had done previously.

Religion and Culture as Lenses for Interpreting Coming Out

For some respondents, there was an additional layer of complexity in relation to their coming out experience—their religion and culture which, in some cases, was perceived or represented by others as incompatible with their sexuality. One respondent reported that others highlighted their "immorality and disobedience to God's demands," viewing them "as some disgrace to the family and God." In short, social norms associated with religion—itself entwined with family identity in some cases—generated emotional distance from valued family members when coming out:

> My parents were very disturbed when I came out to them. For quite some time my mum kept asking me why I chose this path. They came to terms with it now.
>
> They treated me like I was a sinner. They treated me like I was a rebellious child.
>
> Toward the end of my mother's and father's life we no longer spoke. They were not able to accept me for who I am, and thought that my husband and I having a child was an abomination of God.
>
> For a week my mum cried and eventually she asked me if I was still "thinking I was that way" and just to shut her up and keep her out of it I said yes, and that I'm straight and God saved me.

Participants referred to religious pressures from significant others, in some cases leading to emotional distance and loss. The religious representation that one has "chosen this path," that is, to be LGB, was the common thread in participants' accounts of religious pressures when coming out. Individuals were reportedly treated as being "rebellious," "sinners," and even as "an abomination." In order to limit complete loss of the relationship, some feigned heterosexuality, claiming, as one participant did, that God had "saved" them. In view of religious and other social pressures, some family members reportedly construed the coming-out individual's sexual identity as a significant threat to the family and thus one to be concealed from others:

> They seemed to feel that it was all a great secret and drama—which it wasn't—and even now I feel that they make more of the fact than is necessary. They need to move on. It's not an issue so why maintain an attitude that perpetuates a kind of barrier between us.

In this case, the individual's sexual identity was construed as a "great secret and drama," which generated "a kind of barrier." This amounted to emotional distance from the family. Some respondents felt obliged to "return to the closet" having shared their sexual identity with others. Essentially their sexual identity was not acknowledged by significant others. This was attributed to the perception that their religion and culture took precedence over their own identity and wellbeing:

> Religion took priority over our relationship. I came out to my family and lost them because religion was more important.

> My parents could not see beyond our culture so we just became distant and I was on thin ice with them after I told them I'm bisexual.

Some coming-out LGB individuals who felt that their religion and culture had induced emotional distance from their significant others came to reevaluate their own relationship with their religion and culture:

> Christianity. This was a bad thing that happened when I came out to my whole family (big mistake).

> A bad change for me was my loss of religion. I left Islam when my parents became distant because I came out to them. They changed my whole perception of religion because of the way they treated me when I came out to them.

> I was an average Christian but when I came out and I was ignored and kept at arm's length. I realized Christianity had ruined my life and I stopped being a Christian. I am an atheist now.

These extracts indicate that coming-out individuals attributed the negative reactions that they received to their religion. One respondent referred to Christianity as "a bad thing that happened" when he came out to his family which he now considered to have been a "big mistake" in view of his religion. Religion was therefore perceived as a significant barrier to achieving the social and psychological benefits that he had hoped for in coming out to his family. Some respondents reported disidentifying from their religion because they had come to evaluate it negatively, viewing it as the cause of emotional distance from significant others. It is important to note the considerable psychological burden of this emotional distance, which one respondent described as having "ruined my life." Consequently, some coming-out individuals reevaluated the role of religion in their identity ("this changed my whole perception of religion") and, in some cases, removed it from the identity structure ("I stopped being a Christian. I am an atheist now").

Interview Accounts from Lesbian, Gay, and Bisexual People

In this section, the following three themes arising from the thematic analysis of the interview accounts are described: (1) differentiating negative reactions from loss; (2) the impact of loss for cognition, affect, and behavior; and (3) coping with rejection, emotional distance, and loss.

Differentiating Negative Reactions from Loss

Interviewees made a distinction between the experience of facing a negative reaction from a significant other and that of ambiguous loss that sometimes followed coming out to a significant other.

> There were loads of different reactions in my family. I have four brothers and one sister. I could see my sister's face drop and two of my brothers didn't like it much and they made a few comments that told me so, to be fair, but they made it clear that I was still their brother and I was wanted and loved so the reaction wasn't great but at least I wasn't being excluded. My parents were different. They didn't say anything as such but our relationship hasn't been the same since and I get the sense that I'm not their son anymore. It's really heartbreaking that my sexuality has come between us. (Sam, gay man)

> I get that it's a shock at first and I expected that. It's like a clash between their values and mine but you can tell me how you feel but still treat me like I'm "us" rather than like "them" but this is what I got when I came out. I became a pariah because I was sinning in their eyes. (Jill, lesbian woman)

> You'd expect parents to get all angry and everything but mine are basically fine with me. It's my brother. We had a really close relationship but it has gone. It's like he's ashamed of me and what I represent and that really hurts because we would do everything together. I just don't get it. My parents are fine but I've lost my relationship with him. (Chris, gay man)

LGB people tend to face a multitude of initial reactions to their coming out and the attitudes of significant others can and often do improve (see Chap. 6). Although negative reactions have been found to be associated with psychological distress, as noted earlier in this chapter, some LGB people acknowledge that the negative attitudes implied by such reactions are transient and are optimistic that they will improve. As the accounts above indicate, LGB people are often understanding of their significant others who may initially exhibit "shock" or anger and for whom coming out may engender a "a clash between their values and mine." Similarly, Chris felt that it was understandable that his parents should initially express anger. In short, LGB people are realistic and do not always expect a positive initial reaction when they come out to their significant others.

As indicated by several interviewees, it is sometimes possible to perceive love and affection from significant others who initially exhibit a negative reaction which appears to buffer the negative psychological effects of that negative reaction. Sam and Chris contrasted the negative reaction from their siblings who were reportedly disapproving of their sexuality with that of their parents who were conversely more restrained in their verbal reaction. Sam noted that his parents had not made any explicit statements about his sexuality or their feelings toward his coming out but that he perceived a negative change in their relationship and even that he felt as though he was "not their son anymore." This was echoed by Chris who reported losing his relationship with his brother. These accounts signal not only ambiguous loss of their valued family relationships but also loss of a significant element of identity—that of being a son or brother. Similarly, Jill contrasted generic negative reactions from significant others with the sense of exclusion that she experienced from her parents when she came out to them. This challenged her sense of identity by making her feel like a "pariah" because of the perception among her significant others that her sexuality represented a sin.

Across many interviewees' accounts, this sense of exclusion from the family emerged as being one of the most significant psychological challenges associated with their coming out experience:

> I know things will never be the same again. My parents talk to me. I get food. My clothes get washed but that warmth that we had before, that affection, that has all disappeared. It happened overnight basically. As soon as they found out, they gave up on me. (Joe, gay man)

> The hardest thing wasn't the harsh words like "you'll die of AIDS" or "I'll never know the joy of grandchildren." It's the feeling that you're not wanted in the family and that you're overly differentiated, like you stand out like the "failure son." I don't have any relationship with my dad even though we're living under the same roof. It's really hard to get your head round this because I really miss him and the kind of relationship we had before. (James, bisexual man)

The sense of loss was experienced in many different ways. Some interviewees reported a more subtle sense of distance from their significant others while others, such as Joe and James, reported more overt rejection. For Joe, there was a sense of ambiguous loss in that his relationship with his parents was functional but no longer characterized by warmth and affection which were present in the relationship prior to his coming out as gay. Conversely, James experienced more overt rejection from his parents who invoked HIV/AIDS and childlessness as negative sequelae of his bisexuality. These epithets made him feel that he was "not wanted in the family," that is, rejected. These feelings of rejection were perhaps compounded by the fact that he continued to cohabit with his father despite his father's feelings toward him. In both cases, loss appeared to be associated with identity threat. For Joe, the suddenness of the negative change ("it happened overnight") and the perception that the loss was permanent indicated a possible threat to his sense of continuity. Similarly, for James, the epithets by his significant others used to exclude and reject him made him feel excessively distinctive ("you're overly differentiated") and as a failure, suggesting threats to both distinctiveness and self-efficacy.

Some interviewees constructed the rejection and consequential sense of loss that they suffered as a means of active "punishment" for coming out:

> There's like a distance between us. Our conversations are really on the surface and that's it. What's the word? Superficial. "How was your day?" and "Oh, mine was fine" and then we go our separate ways. I've tried mentioning it again and sorting it out but [her cousin] doesn't want to know. I know I'm a big disappointment and she is punishing me for coming out. The funny thing is she always knew but it was just when I decided to tell her clearly—not once but twice—that she retaliated by being really, really cold with me. (Jen, lesbian woman)

> I remember it so clearly exactly what I felt [..] my so-called friend ordered pizza with everyone and blanked me, excluded me from it, because of what I told him two days before so I was basically just treated like a non-person, like blanked totally. It was on purpose to make me feel bad for deciding to be myself, like it's a crime. (Michael, gay man)

In some cases, the preference is simply not to know, that is, to feign ignorance of one's sexuality. Jen's cousin had reportedly always known but refused to acknowledge her sexuality. When Jen came out to her cousin, she continually refused to acknowledge this information and her cousin's insistence—by coming out again—reportedly led to a breakdown in their relationship. Indeed, it has been noted in previous research that LGB people may feel compelled to come out more than once when the information is not assimilated and accommodated by their interlocutor (Denes & Afifi, 2014). Jen perceived this as a form of retaliation.

Similarly, Michael recalled that his former friend to whom he had disclosed his sexual identity deliberately sought to exclude him from their friendship circle subsequent to his coming out. Both accounts highlighted a common characteristic in these experiences of loss—the persons in whom they confided subsequently became distant from them. Conversations became superficial and, in some cases, the coming-out individual's existence was no longer acknowledged. This was clearly distressing for some. Jen sought to restore her relationship with her cousin whom she perceived to be growing increasing distant while Michael no longer considered the person he came out to a true friend.

The Impact of Loss for Cognition, Affect, and Behavior

Rejection, emotional distance, and the consequential sense of loss that some LGB people face can have implications for the ways in which they think, feel, and subsequently behave. The clearly negative implications of coming out to unsympathetic significant others included threats to all four principles of identity.

> I just felt really, really lonely despite actually not being alone. I mean, there were a lot of us around and I was always around people. That was what cut right through me and made me depressed. I just felt like I was worthless and nobody wanted to be near me. Plus the emptiness of our relationship has affected me a lot because I just want the life I had before but that is not going to happen, that's for sure. (Sam, gay man)

> My family are there and my parents are there. It's not like they've disowned me openly but I don't feel like I can depend on them, like count on them anymore. It makes me feel quite lonely, alone, and powerless because I don't feel like I've got their backing, not financial. I mean like their emotional backing. (Sarah, lesbian woman)

Sam described his feelings of intense loneliness despite regularly being in the physical presence of others. This could be attributed to the perception that his significant others were compelled—due to their living arrangements—but did not really wish to be in his presence. His relationship with his family was now characterized by "emptiness." The construal of his family relations in this way attested to his sense of ambiguous loss due to the distance he now perceived from his significant others. This appeared to challenge his self-esteem ("I just felt like I was worthless") as well as his sense of continuity since he longed for, but believed that he could not recover, "the life [he] had before." Similarly, Sarah lamented the loss of her parents' "emotional backing" even though they remained physically present, communicative, and even financially supportive. This made her feel "powerless," since she wished to but felt that she could not ameliorate this situation, suggesting a loss of self-efficacy.

> I think what makes it really hard is the uncertainty like the to-ing and fro-ing because I can tell my relationship with my brother isn't the same as before but sometimes he'll be really nice and the next minute he is cold so it's like I don't know where I stand with him. Yesterday was one thing, today is another and tomorrow might be different. Really I just want some stability back. (Ken, gay man)

Ken described the ambiguous loss due to his family's reaction to his coming out in terms of uncertainty. He felt uncertain because his family's behavior toward him was reportedly inconsistent. At times his brother appeared to accept him, though perhaps not his sexuality, while at others he was distant toward him. Indeed, several interviewees invoked their confusion at the behavior of significant others subsequent to their coming out. For Ken, the inconsistency between past, present, and future ("the to-ing and fro-ing") generated uncertainty which might undermine his sense of continuity between past, present, and future. There was a desire among coming-out individuals who perceived uncertainty to recover some stability. Those who felt that this was impossible sometimes regretted coming out in the first place.

Identity process theory postulates that individuals will seek to maintain and, in cases of threat, restore the identity principles. Indeed, several interviewees noted that they were hesitant about coming out to others and therefore were selective in doing so:

> To be honest, it's sort of made me like wary about coming out to other people because I had to go through a lot of silence, ignoring and that with my family and I am extra cautious about coming out because I'm thinking "will this lead to another problem?" or "will I lose this person forever?" I guess this is what a lot of queer people fear and it's not nice but what we want, what I want, is a bit of predictability to my life and just knowing how you'll be treated. (Deborah, bisexual woman)

> I'm just really careful about who I decide to tell and how much I tell them. I just don't think it's worth it as it's a private me-issue and if it's just going to make me feel like shit and if I'm just going to ruin a good friendship for nothing, what's the point? (Peter, bisexual man)

Emotional distance from significant others that follows coming out may generate not only ambiguous loss in LGB people but also feelings of uncertainty about the future and, more specifically, about how they will be treated by others. Some interviewees were therefore selective in coming out, both in terms of to whom and to what extent they disclosed their sexual identity. In other words, they came to feel cautious about sharing a significant element of their identity, viewing this as "risky" given that their sexual identity might not be understood or accepted by significant others. Deborah alluded to her threatened sense of continuity because she felt uncertain about the future and was therefore unable to connect it to the past and present. Loss was a key tenet of her uncertainty ("will I lose this person forever?"). She hesitated about coming out to others in order to safeguard feelings of certainty and, thus, continuity. Similarly, Peter reported being "really careful" about coming out in an attempt to protect his self-esteem ("if it's just going to make me feel like shit"). After all, the breakdown of significant interpersonal relationships may be perilous not only for continuity but also for one's self-esteem (Scharp & Dorrance Hall, 2017).

Sam described the implications of ambiguous loss for his sense of self-efficacy:

> In a way I feel like this has all impacted my boyfriend quite a lot because I'm pretty clingy and I'm clingy because I don't want to lose him. I don't have what I had with my family anymore and I've actually not got strong friendships either so it makes me depend on him a lot more than I did. I'm

not cool with this because I felt a bit too dependent, like I've lost my independence a bit and he's not totally cool with it either. (Sam, gay man)

Perceived rejection from the family can lead individuals to seek feelings of acceptance, inclusion, and belonging from other sources. In his study of British South Asian gay men, Jaspal (2015) found that some of his participants developed a more intense attachment to, and emotional dependence upon, their romantic partners as they were rejected by their parents and family members. Some came to perceive their romantic partners as their only source of emotional security and therefore experienced intense feelings of distress when their romantic relationship subsequently broke down. In a similar vein, Sam essentially described an insecure (anxious) attachment to his romantic partner, which he attributed to his experience of familial rejection as well as the loss of important friendships. In short, the ambiguous and, in some cases, explicit loss that he experienced led him to become more reliant upon his only remaining source of emotional security—his romantic partner. This was clearly not acceptable to him—he himself described his attachment pejoratively as "clingy" and lamented his perceived loss of independence. Autonomy undoubtedly contributes to one's sense of self-efficacy which appeared to be challenged by the attachment style that he had developed in the aftermath of his coming out.

Coping with Rejection, Emotional Distance, and Loss

Experiences of rejection, emotional distance, and loss were clearly threatening for identity. Interviewees described a range of strategies for attempting to cope with the negative psychological effects of these experiences:

> All of them [her extended family] made it really clear to me that what I was doing was wrong—doing, not being, so not who I actually am but what I was doing, in their eyes—so no, I can't be myself around them. It's always an act and that creates a barrier, like a distance between us, but this is all I can do. If I'm myself, I'm excluded. If I pretend to be straight then I'm in but not really because our relationship is meaningless but I just pretend to be straight basically. (Jen, lesbian woman)

> The best thing for me in these circumstances is just telling them what they want to hear, that I'm not a lesbian. (Sally, lesbian woman)

> Fitting in means acting. I mean, acting straight. Otherwise I'm the black sheep of the family. (Jamie, bisexual man)

Interviewees opted for the strategy of passing as heterosexual in order to minimize the risk of rejection, emotional distance, and loss, and to enhance feelings of belonging in the family. Jen noted that it was clear to her that her extended family would not accept her sexual identity which had of course been the goal of coming out to them. They continued to view her sexuality as an undesirable behavior, rather than as a positive aspect of her identity. Consequently, she and others who reported similar experiences felt misunderstood and rejected by their families. The strategy of passing, employed by all three interviewees, limited the negative feelings of distinctiveness associated with their sexuality but it was clearly suboptimal. Jen noted that she could not be herself with her extended family, suggesting that, although she was no longer overtly rejected, she could not derive feelings of authenticity in their presence and that the emotional distance nevertheless remained. Indeed, she described her relationship with her extended family as meaningless because it was now characterized by pretense. Similarly, Jamie described his compliance with others' expectations as "acting," which echoed the negative consequences for his sense of authenticity. In essence, this was about "telling them what they want to hear"—the precise antithesis of coming out.

Some individuals reported persevering with coming out and attempted to come out a second time in order to claim a sense of belonging in the family in spite of the rejection, emotional distance, and loss that they had experienced the first time. This was essentially an attempt to cope and to derive belonging and authenticity:

> I suppose I went for the "tough love" approach. I came out to my parents and there was like an icy silence for months. They literally wouldn't talk to me. So I brought it up again and basically came out to them twice as in "this is who I am and I'm not changing who I am" to lay it down once and for all. That was sort of like the nail in the coffin because we haven't talked about it and they're not the same with me. I'm on eggshells with them.

> There's this big emotional void now even though we used to have a relationship. (Ken, gay man)

> I tried a few more times. Like they were ignoring me and being difficult. If the opportunity came up, like a guy with another guy who had come out as gay, I was like "oh I know how he feels" to get the conversation going about it but it pushed them further and further away from me and we just ended up on greeting terms and not really having a relationship. They preferred that to talking about my identity and that does make me feel a bit helpless about this all. (Joe, gay man)

> I just gave up in the end. Now it's a no-go area of conversation. I mentioned it a couple of times but realized that this was going nowhere and actually it was just making them distant. We just don't talk about it. It is as if they don't know and I'm at peace with that now because I wake up thinking "yes, new day, I feel good." Before it was like a black cloud over me all the time. It was pretty horrible. (Janet, lesbian woman)

When individuals came out the first time, they were faced with rejection, emotional distance, and loss, which they attempted to address by coming out a second time. They wished to affirm their sexual identity but also to salvage their relationships with significant others. Some did so by forcefully coming out a second time while others employed indirect methods, such as using cues in their social context to raise the question of their sexuality once again. However, the objective of seeking a sense of belonging was not consistently achieved. Indeed, Ken described this as the "nail in the coffin" in his relationship with his parents who subsequently became more distant. He himself felt that he could not be authentic in their presence and remained nervous about discussing certain topics with them: "I'm on eggshells with them."

Similarly, Joe's attempt to come out again resulted in greater emotional distance from his family: "it pushed them further and further away from me." He noted the adverse impact that this had on their relationship which became superficial—his family did not wish to discuss the topic of his sexuality and thus preferred to limit interaction with him. The psychological impact of the rejection, emotional distance, and loss that participants experienced following their attempts to cope (by coming out again) were clearly expressed by these interviewees. This made them question their self-esteem and self-efficacy.

In contrast, Janet decided not to pursue coming out, having attempted to do so repeatedly but to no avail. Her coping strategy consisted of focusing on the positive aspects of the situation, namely that she at least retained a connection with her significant others, on the condition that she avoid the topic of her sexuality. Although this was threatening for her self-esteem, her focus on these positive aspects of the situation alleviated this threat and enabled her to derive psychological wellbeing.

Some interviewees reported avoiding the topic of their sexuality without necessarily passing as heterosexual in order to enhance their relationship with significant others:

> My aim has been to try to salvage what I can from our relationship which has all but broken down so I do really make an effort with my family—all of them—you know, to talk, to be normal and try to show them that I'm actually still the same person and they shouldn't just ignore me. But this hasn't really worked that well since I came out. The trying and failing with my family really affects my mental state because I feel pretty bad about my sexuality. I just feel like I've lost what I had with them and I wonder "was it [coming out] really worth it?" (Ali, gay man)

When LGB people come out, they may be viewed by significant others primarily through the lens of their sexuality. In other words, this aspect of their identity may be foregrounded by others and, when their sexuality is perceived negatively, they too may be viewed negatively and stigmatized. Accordingly, Ali described his attempt to show his parents that he was "still the same person" despite his sexuality, which he believed would enhance his relationship with them. Ali referred to the breakdown of his relationship with his parents who were now ignoring him. Crucially, this had detrimental effects upon his psychological wellbeing. He felt that he had failed in his attempt to improve his valued relationship with his family. Moreover, feelings of rejection, emotional distance, and loss were associated with internalized homonegativity since Ali now questioned the value and worth of his sexual identity. He now doubted the value of coming out to his parents and expressed regret about having done so.

It is important to note that a key motive for coming out as LGB is the quest for acceptance, inclusion, and belonging. Coming-out individuals hope to be understood by their significant others and there is an element of trust that underpins the process. They may experience disappointment and threats to identity when the support they seek does not materialize. While some reported attempting to come out a second time to derive the belonging that they had originally sought in coming out, others essentially gave up and decided to seek interpersonal support from alternative sources:

> My parents were my everything. I remember getting my exam results and walking home and I rang them first. You know, we were real close and did everything together. But they changed because I guess I changed for them when I let them in [came out] and they rejected me because of that. We live together but there's a lot of distance and coldness. I've got a lot closer to my friends and they are more of a family to me now, if I'm honest with you. It's sad but they were there for me and my parents weren't so who is my true family? (James, bisexual man)

> When I came out, I went through a period of grief because I lost everyone around me in my family. I was actively avoiding being at home and started going out on the [gay] scene a lot and made some close friends who, to be fair, have supported me through thick and thin, including in my arguments and the problems with my family. I have that feeling of loss but it's a bit easier knowing I have found my tribe. (Ali, gay man)

Participants powerfully described their feelings of loss when they were rejected by and felt distant from their significant others. James illustrated the significance of his parents in his identity ("my parents were my everything") and recounted the important role that they had played in his life. Moreover, Ali reported experiencing "a period of grief" due to the loss of his relationship with his family after coming out. Coming-out individuals who are rejected by their family may seek feelings of acceptance and inclusion from an alternative "chosen family." James reported becoming closer to his friends whom he described as "more of a family to me now" and, in view of the support that they provided, were now considered "my true family." Similarly, Ali described developing close friendships with other LGB people whom he had met on the gay scene. They reportedly supported him "through thick and thin" especially in relation to the challenges that he had experienced with his family. Although individuals who faced rejection from their families clearly experienced threats to their psychological wellbeing, they could cope to some extent due to the support that they received from others. This provided at least some psychological respite.

Overview

When LGB people contemplate coming out, they are often fearful about facing a negative reaction from significant others. This chapter provides detailed insight into experiences of rejection, emotional distance, and ambiguous loss in the aftermath of coming out to somebody who matters. These negative reactions are particularly insidious because they do not necessarily entail complete abandonment but rather emotional estrangement. Coming-out individuals no longer felt connected to people whom they valued. They described the tension in their relationships and subsequent feelings of loss—both loss of aspects of their relationships with others and loss of the individuals themselves. The risk was heightened when their sexuality was viewed by significant others through the lenses of religion or traditional culture.

Yet, it is important to note that coming-out individuals were generally realistic and pragmatic about their coming out and expected some negative reaction at least in the immediate aftermath of their coming out. They differentiated between initial negative reactions and the more severe types of rejection, emotional distance, and loss described in this chapter. The latter was especially threatening for identity, especially for self-esteem and continuity, and the uncertainty associated with ambiguous loss experiences, in particular, appeared to generate some identity doubt.

Coming-out individuals who faced negative reactions of this kind attempted to cope using varied strategies. Some attempted to come out again in order to reinforce their identity but to no avail. In cases of continued rejection, emotional distance, and loss, some people reported seeking support from an alternative "chosen family," mostly commonly other LGB people, and distancing themselves from their families of origin. Others reported returning to the closet and feigning heterosexuality since they felt that it was futile to attempt to come out again and that to do so would once again imperil valued interpersonal relationships. In short, fears of rejection that commonly precede coming out, often delaying or inhibiting it, were experienced with harmful effects for identity.

References

Ben-Ari, A. (1995a). Coming out: A dialectic of intimacy and privacy. *Families in Society: The Journal of Contemporary Social Services, 76*(5), 306–314. https://doi.org/10.1177/104438949507600504

Ben-Ari, A. (1995b). The discovery that an offspring is gay: Parents', gay men's, and lesbians' perspectives. *Journal of Homosexuality, 3*(1), 89–112. https://doi.org/10.1300/J082v30n01_05

Bird, J. D., LaSala, M. C., Hidalgo, M. A., Kuhns, L. M., & Garofalo, R. (2017). "I had to go to the streets to get love": Pathways from parental rejection to HIV risk among young gay and bisexual men. *Journal of Homosexuality, 64*(3), 321–342. https://doi.org/10.1080/00918369.2016.1179039

Cafferty, J. (2017). *Coming out and losing out: Gay men in emerging adulthood and family support*. M.A. dissertation, University of Arkansas, Fayetteville, USA. https://scholarworks.uark.edu/etd/2504/ [Accessed 1 September 2025]

Carastathis, G. S., Cohen, L., Kaczmarek, E., & Chang, P. (2017). Rejected by family for being gay or lesbian: Portrayals, perceptions, and resilience. *Journal of Homosexuality, 64*(3), 289–320. https://doi.org/10.1080/00918369.2016.1179035

Carbone, A., Pistella, J., Gennaro, A., Petrocchi, C., & Baiocco, R. (2023). Parental experiences of coming out: From "un-doing family bonds" to "family generativity". *Journal of Homosexuality, 70*(10), 2135–2157. https://doi.org/10.1080/00918369.2022.2048334

Chester, M. R., Sinnard, M. T., Rochlen, A. B., Nadeau, M. M., Balsan, M. J., & Provence, M. M. (2016). Gay men's experiences coming out online: A qualitative study. *Journal of Gay & Lesbian Social Services, 28*(4), 317–335. https://doi.org/10.1080/10538720.2016.1221785

Cramer, D. W., & Roach, A. J. (1998). Coming out to mom and dad: A study of gay males and their relationships with their parents. *Journal of Homosexuality, 15*(3/4), 79–91. https://doi.org/10.1300/J082v15n03_04

D'Amico, E., & Julien, D. (2012). Disclosure of sexual orientation and gay, lesbian, and bisexual youths' adjustment: Associations with past and current parental acceptance and rejection. *Journal of GLBT Family Studies, 8*(3), 215–242. https://doi.org/10.1080/1550428X.2012.677232

D'Amico, E., Julien, D., Tremblay, N., & Chartrand, E. (2015). Gay, lesbian, and bisexual youths coming out to their parents: Parental reactions and youths' outcomes. *Journal of GLBT Family Studies, 11*(5), 411–437. https://doi.org/10.1080/1550428X.2014.981627

Davis, K. C., & Anderson, J. L. (2021). The role of perceived parental acceptance-rejection on personality psychopathology in sexual orientation minority young adults. *Journal of Child and Family Studies, 30*(1), 276–291. https://doi.org/10.1007/s10826-020-01858-3

de Lange, J., Baams, L., van Bergen, D. D., Bos, H. M. W., & Bosker, R. J. (2022). Minority stress and suicidal ideation and suicide attempts among LGBT adolescents and young adults: A meta-analysis. *LGBT Health, 9*(4), 222–237. https://doi.org/10.1089/lgbt.2021.0106

DeChants, J. P., Shelton, J., Anyon, Y., & Bender, K. (2022). "It kinda breaks my heart": LGBTQ young adults' responses to family rejection. *Family Relations, 71*(3), 968–986. https://doi.org/10.1111/fare.12638

Denes, A., & Afifi, T. D. (2014). Coming out again: Exploring GLBQ individuals' communication with their parents after the first coming out. *Journal of GLBT Family Studies, 10*(3), 298–325. https://doi.org/10.1080/1550428X.2013.838150

Dorri, A. A., Stone, A. L., Heffington, B. I., Njowo, P. J., Rivera, G., Schnarrs, P. W., & Salcido, R. (2024). "We're not gonna talk about this, it didn't happen. You're confused": Adverse communication in family responses to mental health, childhood sexual assault, and LGBTQ identities. *Society and Mental Health, 14*(1), 39–55. https://doi.org/10.1177/21568693231170901

Dziengel, L. (2015). A be/coming-out model: Assessing factors of resilience and ambiguity. *Journal of Gay & Lesbian Social Services, 27*(3), 302–325. https://doi.org/10.1080/10538720.2015.1053656

Eaton, A. A., & Rios, D. (2017). Social challenges faced by queer Latino college men: Navigating negative responses to coming out in a double minority sample of emerging adults. *Cultural Diversity & Ethnic Minority Psychology, 23*(4), 457–467. https://doi.org/10.1037/cdp0000134

Enderwitz, M., Morgan, V. R., Roberson, A. J., & Schanding, G. T., Jr. (2024). Perceived parental rejection as a predictor of psychological distress in LGBQ+adults and the moderating effects of self-acceptance of sexuality. *LGBTQ+ Family: An Interdisciplinary Journal, 20*(3), 171–189. https://doi.org/10.1080/27703371.2024.2306305

Etengoff, C., & Daiute, C. (2014). Online coming-out communications between gay men and their religious family allies: A family of choice and origin perspective. *Journal of GLBT Family Studies, 11*(3), 278–304. https://doi.org/10.1080/1550428X.2014.964442

Ghosh, A. (2020). After coming out: Parental acceptance of young lesbian and gay people. *Sociology Compass, 14*(1), e12740. https://doi.org/10.1111/soc4.12740

Giano, Z., Currin, J. M., Wheeler, D. L., & Hubach, R. D. (2022). Outness amplifies the negative effect of gay related rejection in rural, but not urban sexual minority men. *Psychology & Sexuality, 13*(2), 240–254. https://doi.org/10.1080/19419899.2020.1765411

Hatchel, T., Merrin, G. J., & Espelage, D. (2019). Peer victimization and suicidality among LGBTQ youth: The roles of school belonging, self-compassion, and parental support. *Journal of LGBT Youth, 16*(2), 134–156. https://doi.org/10.1080/19361653.2018.1543036

Hill, R. M., & Pettit, J. W. (2012). Suicidal ideation and sexual orientation in college students: The roles of perceived Burdensomeness, thwarted belongingness, and perceived rejection due to sexual orientation. *Suicide and Life-threatening Behavior, 42*(5), 567–579. https://doi.org/10.1111/j.1943-278X.2012.00113.x

Jaspal, R. (2012). "I never faced up to being gay": Sexual, religious and ethnic identities among British South Asian gay men. *Culture, Health and Sexuality: An International Journal for Research, Intervention and Care, 14*(7), 767–780. https://doi.org/10.1080/13691058.2012.693626

Jaspal, R. (2015). The experience of relationship dissolution among British Asian gay men: Identity threat and protection. *Sexuality Research & Social Policy, 12*(1), 34–46. https://doi.org/10.1007/s13178-014-0175-4

Jaspal, R. (2020). Parental reactions to British South Asian young men who identify as gay. *Journal of GLBT Family Studies, 16*(4), 402–417. https://doi.org/10.1080/1550428X.2019.1684412

Jaspal, R., & Cinnirella, M. (2010). Coping with potentially incompatible identities: Accounts of religious, ethnic and sexual identities from British Pakistani men who identify as Muslim and gay. *British Journal of Social Psychology, 49*(4), 849–870. https://doi.org/10.1348/014466609X485025

Jaspal, R., & Cinnirella, M. (2012). Identity processes, threat and interpersonal relations: Accounts from British Muslim gay men. *Journal of Homosexuality, 59*(2), 215–240. https://doi.org/10.1080/00918369.2012.638551

Jaspal, R., & Siraj, A. (2011). Perceptions of 'coming out' among British Muslim gay men. *Psychology and Sexuality, 2*(3), 183–197. https://doi.org/10.1080/19419899.2010.526627

Jhang, J. (2018). Scaffolding in family relationships: A grounded theory of coming out to family. *Family Relations, 67*(1), 161–175. https://doi.org/10.1111/fare.12302

Kibrik, E. L., Cohen, N., Stolowicz-Melman, D., Levy, A., Boruchovitz-Zamir, R., & Diamond, G. M. (2019). Measuring adult children's perceptions of their parents' acceptance and rejection of their sexual orientation: Initial development of the Parental Acceptance and Rejection of Sexual Orientation Scale (PARSOS). *Journal of Homosexuality, 66*(11), 1513–1534. https://doi.org/10.1080/00918369.2018.1503460

LaSala, M. C. (2000). Lesbians, gay men, and their parents: Family therapy for the coming-out crisis. *Family Process, 39*(1), 67–81. https://doi.org/10.1111/j.1545-5300.2000.39108.x

Macbeth, A. J., Vidales, C. A., & Vogel, D. L. (2022). Perceived parental religiosity as a predictor of depression and substance use among LGBTQ+ individuals: The mediating role of perceived familial stigma. *Psychology of Religion and Spirituality, 14*(1), 140–147. https://doi.org/10.1037/rel0000411

Manning, J. (2015). Positive and negative communicative behaviors in coming-out conversations. *Journal of Homosexuality, 62*(1), 67–97. https://doi.org/10.1080/00918369.2014.957127

McLean, K. (2007). Hiding in the closet?: Bisexuals, coming out and the disclosure imperative. *Journal of Sociology, 43*(2), 151–166. https://doi.org/10.1177/1440783307076893

Meanley, S., Flores, D. D., Listerud, L., Chang, C. J., Feinstein, B. A., & Watson, R. J. (2021). The interplay of familial warmth and LGBTQ+ specific family rejection on LGBTQ+ adolescents' self-esteem. *Journal of Adolescence, 93*(1), 40–52. https://doi.org/10.1016/j.adolescence.2021.10.002

Meris, D. (2023). Complicated grief and challenges in LGBTQIA+ communities. In R. B. Turner & S. D. Stauffer (Eds.), *Disenfranchised grief: Examining social, cultural, and relational impacts* (pp. 120–137). Routledge.

Pollitt, A. M., Fish, J. N., & Watson, R. J. (2023). Measurement equivalence of family acceptance/rejection among sexual and gender minority youth by disclosure status. *Journal of Family Psychology, 37*(2), 195–202. https://doi.org/10.1037/fam0001056

Rejiester, N. (2014). *Perception of alienation from parents and peers during the coming out process for lesbian, gay, and bisexual individuals and self-reported attachment classifications: A preliminary investigation of the relationship between the attachment system and rejection due to sexual orientation.* PhD dissertation, the George Washington University. https://scholarspace.library.gwu.edu/concern/gw_etds/6395w731z?locale=it

Rickards, T., & Wuest, J. (2006). The process of losing and regaining credibility when coming-out at midlife. *Health Care for Women International, 27*(6), 530–547. https://doi.org/10.1080/07399330600770254

Ryan, C., Huebner, D., Diaz, R. M., & Sanchez, J. (2009). Family rejection as a predictor of negative health outcomes in white and Latino lesbian, gay, and bisexual young adults. *Pediatrics, 123*(1), 346–352. https://doi.org/10.1542/peds.2007-3524

Ryan, W. S., Legate, N., & Weinstein, N. (2015). Coming out as lesbian, gay, or bisexual: The lasting impact of initial disclosure experiences. *Self and Identity, 14*(5), 549–569. https://doi.org/10.1080/15298868.2015.1029516

Samarova, V., Shilo, G., & Diamond, G. M. (2014). Changes in youths' perceived parental acceptance of their sexual minority status over time. *Journal of Research on Adolescence, 24*(4), 681–688. https://doi.org/10.1111/jora.12071

Sand, S. (2015). Coming out, being out: Reconciling loss and hatred in becoming whole. *Psychoanalysis, Culture & Society, 20*(3), 250–266. https://doi.org/10.1057/pcs.2014.18

Scharp, K. M., & Dorrance Hall, E. (2017). Family marginalization, alienation, and estrangement: Questioning the nonvoluntary status of family relationships. *Annals of the International Communication Association, 41*(1), 28–45. https://doi.org/10.1080/23808985.2017.1285680

Sheets, R. L., Jr., & Mohr, J. J. (2009). Perceived social support from friends and family and psychosocial functioning in bisexual young adult college students. *Journal of Counseling Psychology, 56*(1), 152–163. https://doi.org/10.1037/0022-0167.56.1.152

Smith, E. R., Perrin, P. B., & Sutter, M. E. (2020). Factor analysis of the heterosexist harassment, rejection, and discrimination scale in lesbian, gay, bisexual, transgender, and queer people of colour. *International Journal of Psychology, 55*(3), 405–412. https://doi.org/10.1002/ijop.12585

Taylor, A. B., & Neppl, T. K. (2023). Sexual identity in lesbian, gay, bisexual, transgender, and queer or questioning emerging adults: The role of parental rejection, and sexuality specific family support. *Journal of Family Issues, 44*(2), 409–428. https://doi.org/10.1177/0192513X211050063

Thompson, C. A. (1996). Lesbian grief and loss issues in the coming-out process. In C. J. Alexander (Ed.), *Gay and lesbian mental health: A sourcebook for practitioners* (pp. 211–222). Harrington Park Press.

Valdiserri, R. O., Holtgrave, D. R., Poteat, T. C., & Beyrer, C. (2019). Unraveling health disparities among sexual and gender minorities: A commentary on the persistent impact of stigma. *Journal of Homosexuality, 66*(5), 571–589. https://doi.org/10.1080/00918369.2017.1422944

VanBergen, A. M., & Love, H. A. (2022). Family-of-origin rejection on suicidal ideation among a sexual minority sample. *Journal of Marital and Family Therapy, 48*(2), 560–575. https://doi.org/10.1111/jmft.12484

Wheat, L. S., & Thacker, N. E. (2019). LGBTQ+ loss experiences and the use of meaning reconstruction with clients. *Journal of LGBT Issues in Counseling, 13*(3), 232–251. https://doi.org/10.1080/15538605.2019.1627973

Willoughby, B. L. B., Doty, N. D., & Malik, N. M. (2010). Victimization, family rejection, and outcomes of gay, lesbian, and bisexual young people: The role of negative GLB identity. *Journal of GLBT Family Studies, 6*(4), 403–424. https://doi.org/10.1080/1550428X.2010.511085

8

Non-acknowledgement, Invalidation, and Silencing

Negative Interpersonal Repercussions of Coming Out

Although coming out itself has important benefits at the intrapsychic level, as discussed in the previous chapter, there may be negative repercussions for social relationships and, in particular, family relationships (Ford, 2004). In their literature review, Heatherington and Lavner (2008) show that family-level variables, such as family cohesion, closeness and support, and general attitudes in the family, play an important role in how coming out is experienced and managed by lesbian, gay, and bisexual (LGB) people. They propose a model that suggests that the nature of family interactions about LGB issues, as well as interactions in general, following the initial disclosure experience in turn shape self- and other-acceptance and psychological wellbeing in both the coming-out individual and family members. Rejection is a common reaction to coming out and can be manifested in many different ways. This chapter focuses on more subtle forms of rejection, namely through the non-acknowledgement, invalidation, and silencing of the coming-out LGB individual's sexuality.

R. Jaspal, *The Psychology of Coming Out*,
https://doi.org/10.1007/978-3-032-02599-9_8

Rejection sensitivity arises when people "learn to anticipate—indeed expect—negative regard from members of the dominant culture" which in turn makes them vigilant in their interactions with others (Meyer, 2003, pp. 680–681). In their overview of the relevance of the rejection sensitivity model for LGB young people, Baams et al. (2020) note that early experiences of rejection (especially those from valued significant others) can shape the "learning history" of the coming-out LGB person, thereby precipitating rejection sensitivity in future contexts and interactions. Furthermore, they note that rejection experiences in contexts and from people habitually deemed to be "safe," such as one's family members, may reinforce rejection sensitivity. Crucially, people may come to expect and anticipate rejection in contexts in which this is possible but not certain and they may interpret innocuous reactions as rejecting.

Parental rejection and psychological distress are correlated and the relationship between them has been found to be mediated by internalized homonegativity and social support (Puckett et al., 2015). In other words, parental rejection may itself shape the coming-out individual's own perception of their sexuality and lead them to believe they are unsupported, thereby precipitating greater distress. Furthermore, Pachankis et al. (2008) found parental rejection to be associated with sensitivity to future gay-related rejection via internalized homonegativity in a sample of gay men. Both parental and peer rejection in childhood have been found to affect attachment in adulthood in LGB people (Landolt et al., 2004). Moreover, negative parental reactions are associated with poor family functioning (pre-existing dysfunction within the family) and strong beliefs in traditional values, which themselves are shaped by broader social representations (Baiocco et al., 2016).

In their cross-sectional study of 309 LGB people, Carnelley et al. (2011) found that parents perceived by respondents to be accepting and encouraging of their independence reportedly reacted more favorably to their coming out. There appeared to be implications of parental reactions for identity and wellbeing in adulthood—the more favorable the mother's reaction, the less romantic attachment anxiety experienced by the LGB person in the long term. Family rejection has also been found to be associated with future sexual identity concealment, that is, reduced likelihood of coming out to others, possibly due to rejection anticipation

(Salerno et al., 2023). In other words, when parental rejection results in internalized homonegativity it is more likely to generate rejection sensitivity in interactions with others.

Family rejection can deprive coming-out LGB people of the instrumental and social support that they seek when they come out to significant others. Research has found that this can increase engagement in health risk behaviors, such as substance misuse and "survival sex," that is, sex in exchange for food, shelter, and money (Bird et al., 2017). Conversely, a supportive response from significant others, especially one's family, has been shown to affect psychological wellbeing among LGB people. For instance, a longitudinal study showed greater distress at three time points during a 5.5-year period among LGB participants with low or no family support than those with high family support (McConnell et al., 2016). Savin-Williams (2001) notes three barriers to coming out to one's family: (1) a lack of closeness among family members; (2) cultural factors that may lead to the stigmatization of the coming-out individual's sexuality; and (3) fears of serious negative repercussions, such as rejection or even being removed from the family home.

When LGB people come out to significant others, they may feel that the information that they are relaying to them is not being heard. Their coming out may be met with silence or even denial. Denes and Afifi (2014) surveyed 106 LGB individuals about their experiences of coming out to their parents. They found that approximately 25% of participants felt that they had to come out to their parents for a second time, largely to reinforce, clarify, and elaborate on their sexual identity. A second coming out was more likely in cases where the initial coming out experience had been met with feelings of denial from parents. The authors examined the predictors of coming out for a second time and found that, of all the possible reactions to coming out that they examined (i.e., shock, denial, guilt, anger, and acceptance), denial was the only predictor. This suggests that an initial negative reaction is associated with non-engagement with the topic but that denial may generate the perceived need to clarify one's sexual identity with significant others. The authors also found that those who reported a second coming out to their parents reported less satisfaction with their parental relationship, indicating that this had a negative impact on family relations.

In a critical autoethnography, Adams (2014) observes that, among LGB people, their coming out can influence and sometimes even tarnish relationships with significant others. Even after disclosure to a significant other, post-coming out complications can ensue—one's coming out may not be fully acknowledged or understood, for instance. Furthermore, the individual may not be "out" to others within one's broader social circle, potentially putting the coming-out individual and others who already know about their sexual identity in a challenging position. LGB people who face a negative reaction to coming out attempt to cope in varied ways.

Coping

Johnston and Jenkins (2004) conducted an exploratory study of the ramifications of coming out, noting that coming out can disrupt existing relationships with people who believe the coming-out individual to be heterosexual. More specifically, participants in their study described being denigrated by family members as "selfish" for their desire to come out and were therefore advised to remain in the closet. In addition, interviewees described their fears regarding the potential loss of various relationships, including with work colleagues, community members, children (in the case of coming-out parents), and, most commonly, parents and siblings. Individuals were especially fearful that parents and siblings would reject them, and that coming out would compound and aggravate existing tensions in the family.

Some LGB people decide against coming out to significant others because of pre-existing distance in their relationship—they may, for instance, not be on good terms with their parents and therefore see no value in coming out to them (Orne, 2011). In their study of 18 Muslim lesbians, Etengoff and Rodriguez (2022) found that the majority of their participants selectively disclosed their sexuality (i.e., not to everybody) due to fear of familial rejection and that those who noted changes in their familial relationships due to their sexuality reported far higher rates of depression than those who did not. In their analysis of three qualitative datasets, Nordqvist and Smart (2014) found widespread anticipation of hostility from family members and, in some cases, actual experiences of rejection, including family estrangement and the severance of contact. Consequently, some LGB people manage family relationships through "silence, avoidance and non-discussion" (p. 107). All these studies suggest that LGB people tend to take a strategic approach to outness and may limit the extent of their coming out to safeguard valued relationships with others.

Despite rejection from significant others due to sexuality, some LGB people choose to maintain relationships with significant others who reject them because they value these relationships and develop strategies for minimizing the relational impact of their coming out (Echevarria, 2011). The challenge is that individuals in this situation may continually be exposed to psychological stress associated with this distal stressor (i.e., rejection) and proximal stressors (e.g., internalized homonegativity) that can arise from it (Meyer, 2003). Yet, the benefits of maintaining valued relationships may be perceived as outweighing these psychological pitfalls.

The theme of strategic outness is further reiterated in an interview study of 60 Australian bisexual men and women. McLean (2007) found that most participants in their study perceived bisexuality to be misunderstood and stigmatized by others, which led them to "test the waters" in relation to coming out and to be selective in deciding when and to whom to come out. A negative experience can of course shape future willingness to come out. Interviewees in that study did face negative experiences of stigma from significant others when coming out, rendering this a complex decision-making process.

Previous studies have found that coming-out LGB people who face a negative reaction from their family of origin may derive interpersonal support from an alternative family of choice—often friends and other LGB people (Parra et al., 2018). This was also shown in Chap. 7. Notwithstanding the important role of family relations and support in relation to psychological wellbeing in LGB people, there is evidence that peer social support can buffer the impact of negative family attitudes toward one's sexuality on anxiety, as well as the impact of family victimization on depression (Parra et al., 2018). It has also been found that some LGB people may develop families of choice in online contexts to counteract rejection and other identity hazards from significant others when they come out (Etengoff & Daiute, 2014). This can enable them to make sense of the interpersonal challenges as well as reduce their negative impact for psychological wellbeing. Gonzalez et al. (2017) show that extended family members, such as aunts, uncles, and cousins, can also perform this function, contributing to psychological wellbeing among LGB people who face challenges in their relationship with inner family members upon coming out. Moreover, feelings of shame that ensue from parental rejection and detachment following a coming out experience to one's parents can be assuaged through bonding and intimacy with a romantic partner (Kim et al., 2021).

Bry et al. (2017) describe several coping strategies used by LGB people who face familial stigma, including confrontation, acceptance, and forgiveness, focusing on one's future, capitalizing on social support, and building a family of choice to counteract rejection from one's family of origin. Given that parents' own belief and value systems, informed by broader social representations, shape their reactions to their child's coming out as a LGB person, some therapeutic approaches to supporting families to cope with coming out focus on challenging parental beliefs, attributions, and expectations in relation to their child's sexuality (Willoughby & Doty, 2010). The aim is to safeguard the coming-out individual's psychological wellbeing and family relationships.

Written Accounts from Lesbian, Gay, and Bisexual People

In this section, the following three themes arising from the thematic analysis of LGB people's written accounts are described: (1) non-acknowledgement; (2) invalidation; and (3) silencing.

Non-acknowledgement

In addition to loss and emotional distance, which rely upon at least some acknowledgement of the individual's sexuality, there was a strong focus in the data upon non-acknowledgement and silencing:

> I had to come out to my mum a few times because she never "remembered" or acknowledged it.
>
> When I came out to my twin brother things changed between us and we were not as close as we used to be. He refuses to come to my house and he doesn't like being seen out with me in public places. When we are together and it is bought up he will leave the room and completely ignore the situation.
>
> I came out to a girlfriend of mine in high school as bisexual. She ignored any expression of my attraction to men. This caused me to repress said feelings about men for a little bit.

All three participants noted the lack of acknowledgement from their significant others when they came out to them. One respondent reported having to come out "a few times" because the information was not assimilated by their mother. Another described a more passive form of non-acknowledgement—their twin brother would "leave the room and completely ignore the situation" when the topic of sexuality was broached. One individual noted that their friend "ignored any expression" of their bisexuality, leading them subsequently to conceal this element of their identity. Across all three accounts, there was clearly a sense of emotional distance and loss.

Denial is a common strategy for coping with situations with the capacity to threaten identity. Having a significant other come out as LGB can be threatening primarily because it involves change—to relationships and to identity itself (Jaspal, 2020). Moreover, in view of the stigma appended to LGB identities, this change is often deemed to be negative. Some people refuse to assimilate the information being communicated to them. The corpus of participants' accounts provided some insight into the psychological consequences of non-acknowledgement (a manifestation of the denial coping strategy). Some participants came to mirror the denial that they encountered, that is, by repressing their sexuality. This could be attributed to the implicit message that underpins non-acknowledgement, namely that their sexuality is too shameful to acknowledge.

While these constitute relatively passive forms of non-acknowledgement, many respondents described more overt failures of acknowledgement from their significant others:

> She tried to tell me I was confused and now our relationship is not as close as it used to be. I don't know if it ever will be.

> For a brief time, my roommate refused to believe that I was gay. He eventually accepted it, but we aren't friends anymore.

Both participants described others' active attempts to suppress their coming out. People may do this by claiming that the coming-out individual is "confused" which amounts to a form of gaslighting (discussed further in Chap. 9). Non-acknowledgement could have repercussions for the quality of the relationship, leading to emotional distance or even dissolution of the relationship. Furthermore, *refusal* to believe reflects the willful ignorance manifested by some people who simply did not wish to acknowledge the coming-out person's sexual identity.

> My dad suddenly started making a point of talking about how great guys I knew were, and wouldn't it be nice if I was closer with them? Despite flat-out telling him that I was only interested in forming relationships with women (I'm about a Kinsey 5—attraction feelings towards men are just of the "ooh, he's a rare model of a man and nice to look at from a distance" variety).

> Not so much a change, but rather when I first came out my father told me "date however many women you want, but you should only settle down with a man" but eventually I was able to explain how being bisexual works and he eventually came around.

It is possible to acknowledge one's coming out but to interpret this in a way that is more psychologically favorable to the individual who rejects the coming-out person's sexual identity. In the extracts above, participants' fathers reportedly understood and accepted that their offspring had same-sex relationships but labelled these as transient and did not acknowledge them as reflecting a sexual *identity*. Rather they considered it a phase that would eventually pass. Thus, there was a refusal to acknowledge the individual's sexual identity and a tendency to attribute their coming out to some transient phase not to be taken seriously. Moreover, as demonstrated in the extracts above, non-acknowledgement was sometimes coupled with active attempts to bring about change in the coming-out individual's sexuality. One participant noted that her father encouraged her to get "closer" to men while another noted that her father made clear his expectation that she "settle down with a man." These experiences converge in signaling to the coming-out individual that they are not accepted and that their sexuality constitutes a source of shame.

These extracts all reflect attempts from significant others to challenge the individual's sexual identity. They reflect a failure to assimilate and accommodate the information being communicated to them. This may be manifested in many ways: not taking the individual's sexuality seriously; refusal to believe that the individual is LGB; suggesting that the individual is "confused"; and claiming that their sexuality is transient and that eventually they will or should "settle down" with someone of the opposite sex.

Invalidation

In addition to non-acknowledgement, participants' written accounts highlighted a sense of sexual identity invalidation. When sexual minorities share their sexuality with another person, they often hope that the response will be positive and, in particular, that their interlocutor will understand and accept them but also validate their own positive feelings about their sexuality. After all, LGB people tend to come out when they have already reached a degree of self-acceptance at the intrapsychic level (see Chap. 2). Yet, individuals in the sample did not consistently feel understood when they came out, which was particularly the case for those whose significant others appeared to suggest that their sexuality was "a phase":

> People have tended to question whether it is just a phase or a bit of fun because I have always had serious relationships with members of the opposite sex whilst tending to have flings with people of the same sex.

> I had been told "isn't every teenage girl?" as if it didn't matter that I was because so was everyone? Even though I agree people's sexuality is very fluid and everyone is capable of falling in love with the same/different gender, I felt disregarded because it didn't matter to them.

Models of sexual identity development represent the construction of sexual identity as a psychological process that is characterized by doubts in its early stages. Individuals may question whether they are really LGB and sometimes embark upon heterosexual relationships. Similarly, there is growing awareness of the fluidity of sexual identity. Indeed, as noted in the previous subsection, one participant described being "about a Kinsey 5," referring to the Kinsey Scale that measures sexual orientation on a continuous scale (Kinsey et al., 1948). Yet, in the extracts above, these points were reportedly deployed by significant others to invalidate the significance of the coming out event and, more specifically, the coming-out individual's sexual identity. One respondent's father questioned how his daughter could be a lesbian if she had previously had heterosexual relationships with men, while another was told that "every teenage girl" had bisexual tendencies, essentially downplaying the distinctiveness and, thus, significance of her bisexual identity.

> My father gave the typical "it's just a phase, you'll grow out of it" response when I came out. It's meant I'm not as open with him as I could be now.

> After coming out to my mother she told me it was only a phase and did not accept it. I have since been too scared to come out to any other family.

> I came out to my parents at 19. The initial reaction from my mother was okay but it turned out that she commented it was just a phase which hurt a lot.

The extracts indicate that participants' sexuality was not acknowledged as an element of their identity but instead dismissed as a "phase," that is, as a transient behavior. One participant was told that they would "grow out of it," suggesting that their sexuality actually constituted a developmental step or perhaps a symptom of their immaturity. This is antithetical to the sense of identity authenticity discussed in Chap. 5. Furthermore, the extracts provide some insight into the possible psychological and behavioral consequences of receiving a reaction of this kind. The construction of their sexuality as a phase made one participant feel "disregarded." Another felt compelled to "return to the closet," which was similarly noted by others in the sample. One respondent reported that they were now "too scared to come to any other family [member]." It is easy to see how invalidation of one's sexuality in this way can not only undermine psychological wellbeing but also prevent further instances of coming out.

In some cases, there was partial acknowledgement of the individual's sexual identity but not, for instance, of their romantic partner:

> My mother seemed frustrated with the fact I was gay for years after I came out as having a girlfriend. She said it was not normal and always referred to my girlfriend as a friend which made me feel unaccepted.

> When I came out to my father, we suddenly stopped talking about my relationships and we no longer acknowledge or openly discuss anyone that I'm seeing. They are always described as a friend.

When people come out as LGB, they seek acknowledgement and acceptance of their sexual identity, which can include a romantic partner. In the extracts above, individuals' romantic partners were referred to as "a friend"—often accompanied by the desire not to discuss the topic of the coming-out individual's sexual identity. The information that one is LGB may apparently be accepted on a theoretical level but not when the identity is actually enacted, that is, the manifestation of this identity, such as having a same-same partner. This amounts to non-acknowledgement and silencing of one's sexuality. When pressured to acknowledge this and to explicate their actions, significant others made it clear that they felt uncomfortable discussing the topic:

> I think one negative change from coming out to my father, is that the idea of conversations about "who I'm attracted to" are no longer there. It seems to be sort of awkward. However that could just be from a lack of understanding from him.

> My dad made it clear that he accepted me but was uncomfortable talking about it to start with because he didn't understand.

These extracts echo the theme of emotional distance, outlined in Chap. 7. Coming out meant that some topics were off-limits which reduced the scope of discussions and inevitably the scope of one's relationships with significant others. The point is that, for some coming-out LGB people, true validation of their sexual identity would entail discussing with significant others broader elements of it, such as same-sex relationships. This was not always possible. Individuals described how the non-acknowledgement and silencing of their sexual identity made them feel and behave:

> Felt invalidated, never got asked what my sexuality was or what it meant to me, was told it wasn't real.
>
> Told my first boyfriend I was attracted to girls and he said I just wanted to kiss girls to turn guys on. For a long time after that I believed it was true and suppressed my attractions and felt guilty for them.
>
> Being told I am mistaken made me doubt myself because it was coming from someone I thought had my back.

Invalidation appears to be associated with the onset of feelings of identity doubt especially when the source of contradictory information originates from significant others whose opinions and attitudes matter to the coming-out individual. One respondent stated that they personally felt "invalidated" which is in stark contrast to the positive narratives of coming out in which identity authenticity featured prominently. In particular, the veracity of individuals' sexual identity was questioned. In another context of coming out, namely as a bisexual woman to her boyfriend, one participant reported feelings of guilt and suppression because her bisexuality was constructed not as an identity but as a behavior purely for the pleasure of men. The participant's boyfriend appeared to suggest that her coming out was a form of attention-seeking. Indeed, bisexuality may be one of the more contentious sexual identity elements to share since sometimes people, seemingly accepting of gay and lesbian people, contested the veracity of the individual's bisexuality when they came out:

> I have been very careful who I come out to, but many of the times I've come out as bisexual have resulted in the person assuming I'm either "really" gay or straight or disregarding it entirely a few months later, despite my being an adult every time. Often it's met with discomfort as though I was disclosing something inappropriate or a kink.

Following these experiences of non-acknowledgement and silencing, one respondent reported now being "very careful" about coming out as bisexual. Favorable coming out experiences can empower and motivate the individual to share their sexual identity with a greater number of people and to a larger extent. Conversely, the invalidation of their sexual identity made some reconsider their coming out strategy, opting for cautiousness. It is important to note that these acts of non-acknowledgement and silencing also constitute microaggressions, that is, more subtle forms of prejudice that *prima facie* may appear to be more socially acceptable than more overt forms of prejudice, such as name-calling. The fact that, in most cases, the individual's perception of their own identity (or reality) was questioned suggests that this constitutes a form of gaslighting. This is discussed further in Chap. 9.

Silencing

The third dimension of rejection was the active attempt to silence the LGB person's sexuality during and after the coming out event. Participants described various ways in which the information that they communicated to significant others was rejected. In some cases, the extent of their coming out was curtailed and controlled:

> He just changed the subject and I couldn't fully come out to him. It undid all my effort and I didn't discuss it again.
>
> I was just getting ready to tell my mum and she realized and just stopped me mid-sentence and told me not to say something that was going to just change or ruin our relationship and changed the subject.
>
> When I told them, my dad was just quiet and my mum started crying and it made me stop. It felt like a way of stopping the conversation and it made me feel like I was hurting them.
>
> Told to shut up so I never told them ever again. I went back in the depths of the closet.

The individuals who provided these accounts had attempted to disclose their sexual identity to significant others but had been stopped from doing so. They did not encounter an overtly negative reaction to their coming out because in essence they did not feel that they actually had come out. For some, the silencing of their coming out experience led them to refrain from attempting to come out again. The act of being silenced signaled to them that coming out was unadvisable and that it would be best to avoid the subject altogether. This conclusion should be viewed in the context of the significant step that the decision to come out to significant others often constitutes for LGB people. This is rarely a spontaneous decision but rather a process whereby LGB people initially "tests the waters" by coming out to friends and acquaintances before building up the courage to come out to more significant figures in their lives. In some cases, being silenced "undid" the process of building up the courage to come out and placed individuals back "in the depths of the closet."

Being silenced can have broader implications for identity processes. Some individuals appended additional meanings to being LGB based upon their experience of being silenced. Although they were not explicitly denigrated for their sexuality, some reported being made to feel that they were damaging their relationship with their significant others by coming out. As above, one participant was told directly by their mother not to do something (i.e., come out) "that was going to just change or ruin our relationship" and another interpreted her mother's emotional reaction to her coming out as evidence that, by doing so, she was "hurting them." They came to associate coming out with family pain and rupture and, in some cases, decided never to mention the topic again. Indeed, some participants reported that their family members knew that they were not heterosexual and were willing to accept this information passively provided it were never openly acknowledged and discussed. Some family members attempted to maintain the status quo by silencing the topic when attempts were made to discuss it.

For some respondents, coming out was perceived to have disrupted their relationship with their significant others:

> We've always had a special connection and she has always known who I really am but she just can't hear the words "I am gay" and each time we talk about anything to do with this she just changes the subject and this is really frustrating because I haven't had a coming out experience with her because she just shuts me up.

Coming out can be especially challenging for the individual's sense of continuity. After all, the coming-out individual risks a potential rupture with the past and uncertainty about the future. For their significant other, being gay was unacceptable and the means of managing the situation was simply to silence the topic. This deprived the individual of the opportunity to come out to people who matter to them and thus to construct a sexual identity that could be recognized (and validated) by significant others.

> My mother stopped me from telling my dad and told me afterwards that she accepted me and still loved me but that my dad wouldn't so it was best not to tell him anyway. This made me feel bad about myself.
>
> My family basically choose who in my family can and cannot know about my sexual orientation. It is as if I have a gagging order against me. They told me that them accepting me depended on that so they put a condition on my acceptance. It was quite a controlling behavior because my coming out became about them and not me.
>
> I was planning to tell some of my extended family about it but my parents kept interrupting me and making excuses. They did everything within their power to stop me from telling anyone outside my immediate family that I'm a lesbian. So mixed messages. Do they accept me or not?
>
> I felt like I was being given an ultimatum when I came out. Keep quiet and we're OK. Don't and we're not. I felt pressured and quite afraid.

Respondents highlighted another form of silencing in relation to their coming out experience, namely being told by a significant other that, while they themselves accepted the coming-out individual, they disapproved of wider disclosure of their sexual identity. Having accepted their sexual identity at the intrapsychic level, LGB people take the step of sharing this with people that matter to them and whose views are significant. This can provide a sense of support that subsequently enables them to share their sexual identity with a larger number of people and to a greater extent. In short, the support that they perceive from their significant others can have an empowering effect, spurring greater outness. Participants were told that they were accepted, but the fact that their coming out was curtailed by the very same people that purportedly accepted them signaled that their acceptance was conditional: “Keep quiet and we’re OK. Don’t and we’re not.” In some cases, this curtailment was more overt, as some coming-out individuals were advised that “it was best” not to tell other people. One felt that there was a “gagging order” against them, and that significant others did their utmost to limit their outness.

The psychological effects of being silenced in this way were manifold. Some individuals clearly felt that their self-esteem was adversely impacted (“this made me feel bad about myself”), partly because this indicated to them that their sexual identity was a source of shame, not only for them but also for their family. For others, this silencing behavior induced feelings of confusion, uncertainty, and fear since they were told that they were, but did not necessarily feel, accepted. The conditionality of their acceptance made some people feel pressured to adhere to the prescription to remain in the closet. After all, that was essentially what was being asked of them. Individuals were made to feel that they would be accepted provided their coming out remained at a level acceptable to their significant others: within “my immediate family.” Individuals may experience a loss of personal control over their coming out and believe that it is being controlled by others. In short, the LGB person’s coming out—a deeply personal experience—may be appropriated by others.

Interview Accounts from Lesbian, Gay, and Bisexual People

In this section, the following three themes arising from the thematic analysis of participants’ interview accounts are described: (1) playing a role; (2) undoing identity work; and (3) threats to coherence.

Playing a Role

When the coming-out individual is faced with a threat to identity upon coming out, they may engage in compliance, that is, act in accordance with the expectations of others, in order to assuage the threat to identity. This was clearly demonstrated by some interviewees:

> My mother made it really clear to me that she didn't want a gay son. She didn't say as much but it was like really clear to me that she was making me choose. It was really weird because she didn't like say it outright but it was all the ignoring that went on, basically of what I was saying that was like saying "I don't need this right now or ever" so I just acted in line with that afterwards. (Ali, gay man)

Interviewees described the silence surrounding their coming out experience, noting that they were not necessarily denigrated for coming out but that it was simply not acknowledged: "it was all the ignoring that went on." Non-acknowledgement of this kind generated uncertainty because individuals were not explicitly told that their sexual identity was unacceptable but rather they observed undesirable changes in their interpersonal relationships with others and in their behavior toward them. Crucially, these were people to whom they had decided to come out and by whom they hoped to be supported. One interviewee deduced that his sexual identity was unacceptable and felt pressured to "choose" between his sexuality and the one that was deemed preferable by his mother. He concluded that his mother "didn't want a gay son" so he decided to comply with this expectation at least in his self-presentation to her. Similar approaches to identity management were echoed by others:

> I told him [his brother] but he didn't want to know so I never mentioned it again and just went back to how things were, talking about girls, pretending I'm straight. It was craziness because we were both playing dumb and I even started to doubt if we'd ever even had the conversation in the first place. I was playing a game and he was playing along. (Bill, gay man)

> This is what my family want [a heterosexual son] so I'm just playing a role like in a film, but it's a film that they've directed even though this is my life and it takes its toll on you and your feelings because you just, I just felt like I was doing something terrible, as if I was ruining their film. (Ken, gay man)

Interviewees recognized that their significant others were disapproving of their sexual identity. They faced a dilemma—either to pursue coming out and risk the relationship with their significant other or to act in accordance with others' desires. As noted above, Bill described attempting to come out to his brother, facing non-acknowledgement, and opting never to mention the topic again. Furthermore, given the disapproving reaction he faced, Bill decided to feign heterosexuality, as he had done previously, in order to recuperate the past relationship he had had with his brother. In other words, he was fearful that his coming out could disrupt the relationship. This reflected an attempt to maintain a sense of continuity, especially as coming out entails change and, in this case, could risk bringing about negative change in his relationship with his brother. There was, however, a clear downside to this coping strategy: Bill himself acknowledged that he and his brother were "playing dumb" and construed the situation as "craziness." This suggested a potential loss of authenticity in the relationship since both of them knew and recalled that the coming out event had indeed taken place.

Several interviewees described this as "playing a role" and, like Ken, used powerful metaphors for describing their experiences. Ken used a series of cinematic metaphors to communicate the loss of authenticity that he experienced in relation to the compliance coping strategy. He likened his life to a film but one that was being directed by his family members, rather than by himself. Not only did this signal a potential loss of authenticity but also a loss of self-efficacy—Ken no longer felt in control of his life. Several others similarly described the psychological and emotional implications of the compliance strategy. Although they were compliant with the desires of significant others, interviewees noted that this made them feel that they were "doing something terrible" and, in some cases, experienced feelings of guilt due to their sexuality.

> Being with my mates who all know about me it's like a boost to my trueness as a person but then being with my family is like I'm not being my best self here or even my true self and that feels like with coming out it was two steps forward but talking to my family and being around them it's like 100 steps backwards. (Ali, gay man)

Ali described the negative effects of compliance for his sense of authenticity in relation to his family. He construed the concealment of his identity, necessitated in order to comply with familial expectations, as "not being my best self [...] or even my true self." Furthermore, in view of the psychological and emotional steps taken to share their sexual identity with others, this can feel like "progress" for the LGB person: "with coming out it was two steps forward." In other words, this contributes to the development of sexual identity. This was illustrated in reference to Ali's feelings about his identity in the presence of his friends who were reportedly aware and accepting of his sexual identity: "it's like a boost to my trueness as a person." Conversely, the need to engage in the compliance strategy appeared to arrest sexual identity development. Indeed, Ali noted that the concealment of his identity, having taken the decision to come out, constituted "100 steps backwards." This represented a potential threat to continuity, that is, a rupture between his past hopes and expectations of being out, his present reality of complying with familial expectations, and his future uncertainty about the status of his sexual identity in relation to his family.

Yet, it should be acknowledged that some participants who reported engaging in compliance did so as a pragmatic strategy for managing their relationships with others, suggesting that this strategy, though challenging, was preferable to the alternative of pursuing coming out:

> I think you've got to read the room a bit and if it is hurtful then you just avoid that situation and I do that by not talking about my sexuality. They don't ask any questions or anything and I don't tell them anything either. Even in the language I use, it's always like "I'm seeing a friend" and not "I'm meeting a guy to fuck from Grindr" obviously. That's an extreme example (laughs) but you know what I mean right? I'm just telling them what they want to hear and not oversharing what they don't. Things just work for me. (Joe, gay man)

> It's just better this way. Yes, it's not ideal and it's a lot of energy to lie, hide and all that but then I just think at least I've still got a home and I've still got a family that loves me even if they don't completely know me. The odd thing is that they don't know the real me or what they think is the real me because God knows what they're thinking. They just don't admit it. (Sarah, lesbian woman)

> I don't have to deal with the attacks, microaggressions, character assassination and all the rest of it. I can stay relatively sane. It doesn't hurt as much as the silent treatment before. (Jim, bisexual man)

Compliance was construed as a pragmatic approach to the non-acknowledgement, invalidation, and silencing of one's sexual identity. For Joe, it entailed "just telling them what they want to hear and not oversharing what they don't." On the one hand, interviewees noted the psychological pitfalls of the compliance strategy. It was, for instance, acknowledged that the concealment of one's sexual orientation required much mental energy and, as noted earlier in this chapter, the potential loss of authenticity in relation to the family. On the other hand, individuals could at least evade identity hazards associated with their sexuality, such as "attacks, microaggressions, character assassination" and the need to answer difficult questions. LGB people may be better positioned to retain a sense of self-esteem by reducing their exposure to these identity hazards, as well as a sense of continuity by maintaining relationships with significant others which might otherwise be compromised by coming out. The disadvantages of compliance were deemed preferable to the potential threats to identity associated with exposure to these identity hazards. However, like Sarah, some interviewees did acknowledge the negative effects of compliance on their sense of interpersonal authenticity: "the odd thing is that they don't know the real me or what they think is the real me."

Undoing Identity Work

Models of sexual identity development describe the significant "identity work" undertaken in order to come out to others (see Chap. 2). The non-acknowledgement, invalidation, and silencing of the coming-out individual's sexual identity led to the undoing of some of this identity work:

> Honestly I feel helpless and useless because I was being really clear but they were not understanding me and it was intentional. I say I'm a lesbian and no reaction as if they were deaf or I was speaking another language but

> there was no listening involved and that really made me doubt my whole existence. Am I invisible? It sounds stupid but that's the effect it has on you when you're not listened to about something that is pretty damn important in your life. (Janet, lesbian woman)

Having accepted her sexuality at the intrapsychic level, which she herself construed as an important element of her identity, Janet chose to share it with her family. However, upon disclosing her sexual identity to her parents, she reportedly experienced "no reaction" and a lack of listening and understanding, which she attributed to willful ignorance on their part. They simply did not wish to assimilate the information being communicated to them. The effects for her identity were clearly illustrated. On the one hand, she reported feeling "helpless and useless," indicating a potential threat to her self-efficacy. She no longer felt in control and competent. Moreover, she elaborated that the reaction that she encountered caused to her to doubt her identity. This was echoed by another participant:

> It [non-acknowledgement] just makes you doubt a lot in your life and even myself, I was doubting myself and just not understanding whether I was coming or going. (Mike, bisexual man)

Mike's attempt to come out as bisexual to his parents was rebuffed and his sexual identity was not acknowledged. He appeared to experience uncertainty and confusion in relation to his identity. Incidentally, it has been observed that the process of disclosing a bisexual identity, in particular, may be especially challenging from a psychological perspective, as it may be misunderstood (sometimes willfully) and invalidated by others (Hayfield et al., 2018). It must be reiterated that, for many LGB participants, this reflected a retrogression in the identity work that they had undertaken. They had made efforts to reach a point at which they could come out, but felt that they now had to recoil:

> When I thought about telling my family I knew it was going to be tough but I had a plan like I'd tell them and then things would fall into place but it wasn't as I planned it at all because they just didn't want to know and that

made me stuck where I was because I couldn't advance. You know what I mean? It was like being stuck in that dark hole of self-hating or hating that part of myself. I guess I wanted them to support me but they ignored me. (Sarah, lesbian woman)

Coming-out LGB people hope that, despite initial challenges, the overarching objective of achieving acceptance and inclusion will be realized. For some participants, the non-acknowledgement of their sexual identity generated an impasse in identity. As highlighted in the extract above, Sarah felt "stuck where [she] was" that she "couldn't advance" in the ways in which she had planned. She and others hoped that by disclosing their sexual identity to others they would be accepted and supported and, crucially, that they would be able to enact their sexual identity. Yet, the non-affirmative reaction that Sarah actually encountered undermined feelings of self-esteem, clearly demonstrated by her reference to "self-hating" and "hating that part of myself." Internalized homonegativity has been found to be negatively correlated with coming out to others (Jaspal, 2025a, 2025b). It was clear from Sarah's reflections that the non-affirmative reaction from her significant others reinforced the negative self-schema of internalized homonegativity, undoing at least some of the work she had undertaken to disclose her identity to them. The issue of internalized homonegativity was especially noteworthy among interviewees from religious families:

> I grew up in a pretty religious family and so coming out was a big personal journey first as in the self-acceptance was a big thing for me because first I was like "oh I'm sinning" and for a lot of years and then finally I thought "yes, this is who I really am" and if my religion doesn't accept it then too bad for them. But then when you get that reaction like your family aren't hearing you or willing to listen to you then it feels like a lot of that tough stuff was for nothing, I mean, the self-acceptance and then you go back in time to that dark place in the past. (Ali, gay man)

> My attempt to come out was a massive disaster because they just told me it was a phase and I reckon when you hear something enough times from different people all with the same religious agenda it does affect you quite a bit and you start to doubt yourself and I was doubting who I really was.

> I went through the "this is a phase" phase because of my faith and, yes, I found myself going through it again and again because of my family's ignorance and that really hurt. (Ken, gay man)

Interviewees generally described the psychological significance of self-acceptance (at the intrapsychic level) and coming out (at the interpersonal level), both of which formed part of their overall "personal journey" in relation to their sexuality. Participants of religious faith reported the feelings of identity doubt that they had previously experienced (e.g., "I'm sinning" and "you start to doubt yourself"), which they attributed to pressures associated with their religion. Over time, they had succeeded in resisting religious pressures in order to derive self-acceptance and to disclose their sexual identity to significant others. This had not been an easy process. Indeed, research shows the important effects of religion upon psychological coherence and in turn upon willingness to come out to others (Jaspal & Siraj, 2011).

Crucially, interviewees described how a dismissive reaction from significant others (i.e., "your family aren't hearing you or willing to listen to you" and "my family's ignorance") undid the efforts that they had made to overcome religious pressures, and to assimilate and accommodate their sexuality in the identity structure. Their significant others' invalidation of their sexual identity appeared to reignite past feelings of self-doubt and, in the case of Ali, compelling him to "go back in time to that dark place in the past." Similarly, others noted that they came to relive the identity doubt and threat that they had previously experienced when attempting to reconcile their religion and sexuality.

As shown in this chapter, LGB individuals may not necessarily be overtly denigrated but rather their sexual identity may be (subtly) dismissed, invalidated, or silenced. Nevertheless, this can bring about negative psychological consequences, including regression to a past state of identity doubt and threat. This effect may be accentuated among LGB people of religious faith who may, once again, feel the psychological pressures of their religion. In short, the silence of significant others in the face of coming out may signal to LGB individuals that their sexual identity is unacceptable and, in the case of those of religious faith, that it remains and always will be *religiously* unacceptable and irreconcilable.

In disclosing their sexual identity to others, LGB people attempt to enact their identity. They may feel impeded and, in some cases, controlled by significant others when their attempts to come out are resisted:

> I think an important part of the process is telling other people and it's people I choose to tell but with my family like forcing me to stay in the closet then it's like a massive challenge to the type of person I want to be and what I want to tell people. I feel a bit controlled even though I know this isn't their intention really. They don't want to control me, it's just that sexuality issue but they are controlling me and that's the point here. (Sarah, lesbian woman)

In her account, Sarah highlighted the significance of coming out as part of her process of sexual identity development. Yet, the dismissive reaction that she encountered from her family felt like coercion: "my family are forcing me to stay in the closet" and "they are controlling me." This may be threatening for the self-efficacy principle of identity since individuals lack feelings of control and competence over the situation. Furthermore, as indicated by Sarah, a dismissive reaction from a significant other to one's coming out may also challenge one's "ideal self," that is, the identity that one aspires to achieve, in this case, by coming out to others. Sarah indicated that she could not realize her ideal self because her family's reaction was not supportive of her sexual identity: "the type of person I want to be."

There were other ways in which coming-out individuals reported feeling silenced by their significant others:

> My parents told me they loved me but made me promise I wouldn't tell our extended family so I was having to basically pretend when I was with them. It takes a lot of mental energy but it also made me feel like they were ashamed of me and then I started feeling ashamed of myself and those feelings of hating myself for that started creeping in. I found that pretty hard but now I'm OK because I just distanced myself from my uncles and aunts. (Jim, bisexual man)

Reiterating a recurrent theme in participants' written accounts of their coming out experiences, several interviewees acknowledged that their parents initially appeared to accept their sexuality and to respond favorably to their coming out but that they placed other pressures upon them. As noted by Jim, his parents pressured them to conceal his sexuality from extended family members and essentially to "pass" as heterosexual while with them. This signaled to some coming-out individuals that parental acceptance was dependent upon their compliance with this instruction, which has been referred to as conditional acceptance (Sumerau et al., 2018). Moreover, it reflected a form of silencing. Passing was not only psychologically taxing ("it takes a lot of mental energy") but also induced feelings of shame because the requirement to conceal and pass indicated to coming-out individuals that their parents too were ashamed of them. Furthermore, as Jim indicated, this silencing (and partial acceptance of his sexuality) reignited past feelings of shame and self-hatred that he thought he had overcome. Several interviewees indicated that they had since recovered feelings of self-acceptance but that, in order to do so, they had felt the need to distance themselves from family members.

Threats to Coherence

It has been shown that the non-acknowledgement, invalidation, and silencing of their sexuality can have significant effects upon the identity work undertaken by LGB people in preparing to come out to significant others. An especially important psychological effect described by several interviewees was that of threatened psychological coherence. They themselves came to feel that their sexuality was at odds with another important element of identity. This was clearly demonstrated in accounts from interviewees of religious faith:

> For me the big issue has always been about how I can be gay and a Christian at the same time and the truth is I was looking for some guidance from my family but you know the whole eggshells silence around the issue just made that worse for me and I just felt like a failure as a Christian and really like I was sinning. Their silence basically just confirmed that. (Ken, gay man)

> Islam and homosexuality are at odds and I'm still stuck with that. I'm not saying it as if it's something that other people say but it's what I think deep

> down. My parents tolerate me but they don't accept me. If they did accept me then they'd at least show that they hear me but that doesn't happen. We haven't talked about it for 10 years but I can see it in their eyes, it disgusts them. (Ali, gay man)

It has been shown in previous research that significant others can accentuate threats to psychological coherence in relation to sexuality and religion by highlighting explicitly the inconsistencies between these identity elements and "otherizing" LGB people of religious faith (Jaspal & Siraj, 2011; Kashubeck-West et al., 2017). In their accounts, participants also described more subtle threats to psychological coherence.

Some indicated that they sought from their significant others reassurance that it was possible to be LGB and of religious faith (in the case of Ken, gay and Christian) and that they remained accepted despite their sexuality. They wanted to hear from their significant others that their sexual identity was acknowledged and accepted and that it did not compromise their religious identity. Indeed, the identity elements of religion and sexuality can become inter-connected and then engender threats to psychological coherence due to social representations disseminated by people who matter (Jaspal & Cinnirella, 2010). Ken was in the process of attempting to resolve threats to psychological coherence. Yet, his family's silence ("the whole eggshells silence around the issue") appeared to accentuate the threats to psychological coherence that he was experiencing and reinforced his feelings of "failure as a Christian." The perception that one is sinning due to one's sexuality is a common illustration of threatened psychological coherence.

As indicated by Ali, this is also true of some LGB people who identify as Muslim. He indicated that his parents did not "hear" him when he attempted to raise the topic of his sexuality, which seemed to indicate that they were not accepting of it. Several interviewees struggled to interpret the silence of their significant others and generally attributed negative meanings to it, in some cases, deducing that their sexuality caused disgust. In the case of Ali, the silence had persisted for many years and appeared to reinforce, over time, the threat to his psychological coherence. Indeed, he believed that his sexuality and religion were "at odds" and stated that he was "still stuck with that." In short, Ali sought support from significant others to resolve the threat to psychological coherence but encountered silence.

It was clear from participants' accounts that non-acknowledgement, invalidation, and silencing generated feelings of uncertainty. They were not entirely certain about their significant others' views, attitudes, or feelings in relation to their sexuality. They struggled to append meaning to the dismissive reaction to their coming out but generally deduced from it that they were not accepted:

> They carried on asking me when I was going to get myself a girlfriend and get married and have kids and all that and reading between the lines it was their way of saying "if you're gay you're not really a member of this family" and I've always felt like an outsider in that family anyway and this has carried on even though officially I came out to them. Officially I did but they ignored it and act like nothing happened. (Joe, gay man)

Joe exemplified the non-acknowledgement of his sexual identity by describing his attempt to come out to his parents who continued to ask him when he was going to find a girlfriend, get married, and have children with her. He disclosed his identity to them but "they ignored it and act like nothing happened." His parents clearly did not assimilate the information that he communicated to them. For Joe, this demonstrated that, as a gay man, he was not accepted by his family, which undermined his feelings of belonging. However, it symbolized more than a lack of acceptance—his sexual identity and his family identity became interconnected and, as a result of his family's non-acknowledgement, he was made to feel that these identity elements were incompatible. In short, he could not simultaneously be gay and an accepted member of that family. Like the participants of religious faith who perceived long-standing inconsistencies between their sexuality and religion, he had long questioned his position within his family in view of his sexuality ("I've always felt like an outsider anyway"). The psychological estrangement from family identity was similarly illustrated by other interviewees, such as Ali:

> My family brought me up with one particular worldview, like you get married, you have kids and that's that and the fact that my dad is so awkward

> with me whenever I mention anything that's to do with my sexuality says a lot. He doesn't really see me as his son or one of them and so I'm like this outcaste. I just don't see my sexuality as being something that he can accept and because he has so much influence over everyone nobody talks about it or accepts it. (Ali, gay man)

Ali described a very similar situation to that of the previous interviewee. His family and, in particular, his father had a particular worldview: "you get married, you have kids and that's that." As a gay man, he felt that he did not meet these basic criteria for membership in the family, which led him to believe that his father "doesn't really see me as his son or one of them." The latter observation was particularly noteworthy. Ali referred to his family as "them" and explicitly stated that he felt like "this outcaste." This perception of "otherness" suggested that his family identity and sexuality were incompatible and that, as a gay man, he would not be fully accepted, included, or integrated in the family. It is important to note that, as in the accounts of several other interviewees, rejection was not overt but rather *indicated* by the invalidation of his sexuality. In other words, Ali was not overtly denigrated but made to feel that his sexuality was not valid and, thus, not acceptable.

> I can't say they've ever told me I'm a sinner or anything like that but there's something I can't pinpoint that tells me that being gay isn't fully accepted and isn't going to be in our family so I'm a constant outsider and I feel like my life isn't compatible with theirs so there's that kind of conflict for me. I do want to be part of my family but I don't feel like I am. (Ken, gay man)

Similarly, Ken indicated that there was no overt denigration of his sexual identity but rather "something I can't pinpoint" that signaled to him that it was not acceptable to his family. His sexual identity was simply not acknowledged despite his attempts, on several occasions, to come out. Like many other interviewees, the invalidation of his identity in this way made him feel like "a constant outsider" in his family. He yearned to, but did not feel that he did, belong. The main impediment to belonging was his sexual identity which he did not deem to be compatible with his family identity. The threat to psychological coherence was described in terms of an internal conflict.

Some interviewees also described feelings of invisibility due to the non-acknowledgement, invalidation, and silencing that they encountered:

> The more invisible I was becoming in my family, the more shame I was feeling and that shame isn't really good for the pride that I was supposed to be feeling and that for a bit I did feel actually. The two just don't go together. The shame kills the pride and I started to get depressed and just felt like they wouldn't notice if I just moved out one day. (Ali, gay man)

It is possible that "becoming invisible" may constitute a short-term strategy for coping with the threat to psychological coherence in relation to family identity and sexual identity. After all, if the individual is not visible, they can be inconspicuous and the inconsistencies between identity elements may not be flagged by others. Yet, the threat to psychological coherence was clearly felt by Ali who noted a conflict between the feelings of pride that he had begun to derive in relation to his sexual identity and those of shame associated with his family. Invisibility was not deemed to be effective in restoring feelings of psychological coherence but further accentuated his feelings of shame.

Overview

This chapter provides insight into some of the more subtle ways in which coming-out LGB people experience rejection from significant others. In both their written and interview accounts, individuals described facing non-acknowledgement, invalidation, and silencing of their sexual identity when coming out. On the one hand, exposure to these identity hazards appeared to induce identity doubt and identity threat, with several principles of identity being undermined. Some came to feel that their sexuality was inconsistent with other elements of identity, such as their religion and family, precipitating a threat to their sense of psychological coherence. Coming-out individuals who reported feeling rejected in this way attempted to cope in varied ways. Some reported playing a role in order to comply with the perceived expectations of others. They essentially attempted to safeguard valued relationships with others, which they felt were imperiled by coming out. On the other hand, some reported an "undoing" of the identity work that they had undertaken in order to take the significant step of coming out to people who mattered to them. LGB people who take the decision to come out tend to have achieved the assimilation-accommodation of their sexuality in identity and to evaluate it favorably. A negative reaction to their coming out, such as non-acknowledgement, invalidation, and silencing, from significant others may have regressive effects upon their sexual identity development, leading individuals to express doubts about it, to experience internalized homonegativity, and, in some cases, to return to the closet.

References

Adams, T. E. (2014). Post coming-out complications. In R. M. Boylorn & M. P. Orbe (Eds.), *Critical autoethnography: Intersecting cultural identities in everyday life* (pp. 62–74). Routledge.

Baams, L., Kiekens, W. J., & Fish, J. N. (2020). The rejection sensitivity model: Sexual minority adolescents in context. *Archives of Sexual Behavior, 49*(7), 2259–2263. https://doi.org/10.1007/s10508-019-01572-2

Baiocco, R., Fontanesi, L., Santamaria, F., Ioverno, S., Baumgartner, E., & Laghi, F. (2016). Coming out during adolescence: Perceived parents' reactions and internalized sexual stigma. *Journal of Health Psychology, 21*(8), 1809–1813. https://doi.org/10.1177/1359105314564019

Bird, J. D. P., LaSala, M. C., Hidalgo, M. A., Kuhns, L. M., & Garofalo, R. (2017). "I had to go to the streets to get love": Pathways from parental rejection to HIV risk among young gay and bisexual men. *Journal of Homosexuality, 64*(3), 321–342. https://doi.org/10.1080/00918369.2016.1179039

Bry, L. J., Mustanski, B., Garofalo, R., & Burns, M. N. (2017). Resilience to discrimination and rejection among young sexual minority males and transgender females: A qualitative study on coping with minority stress. *Journal of Homosexuality, 65*(11), 1435–1456. https://doi.org/10.1080/00918369.2017.1375367

Carnelley, K. B., Hepper, E. G., Hicks, C., & Turner, W. (2011). Perceived parental reactions to coming out, attachment, and romantic relationship views. *Attachment & Human Development, 13*(3), 217–236. https://doi.org/10.1080/14616734.2011.563828

Denes, A., & Afifi, T. D. (2014). Coming out again: Exploring GLBQ individuals' communication with their parents after the first coming out. *Journal of GLBT Family Studies, 10*(3), 298–325. https://doi.org/10.1080/1550428X.2013.838150

Echevarria, A. E. (2011). *"Because she's my mom": An exploratory study of adult lesbian women's understanding and management of relationships with mothers who reject their sexuality.* Masters thesis, Smith College. https://scholarworks.smith.edu/theses/1062/

Etengoff, C., & Daiute, C. (2014). Family members' uses of religion in post–coming-out conflicts with their gay relative. *Psychology of Religion and Spirituality, 6*(1), 33–43. https://doi.org/10.1037/a0035198

Etengoff, C., & Rodriguez, E. M. (2022). "I feel as if I'm lying to them": Exploring lesbian Muslims' experiences of rejection, support, and depression. In C. Etengoff & E. M. Rodriguez (Eds.), *The LGBTQ+ Muslim experience* (pp. 95–121). Routledge.

Ford, V. E. (2004). Coming out as lesbian or gay: A potential precipitant of crisis in adolescence. *Journal of Human Behavior in the Social Environment, 8*(2–3), 93–110. https://doi.org/10.1300/J137v08n02_06

Gonzalez, J. M., Sinclair, K. O., D'Augelli, A. R., & Grossman, A. H. (2017). Intersectionality and well-being among racial/ ethnic minority and LGB youth: Extended family members as support against negative parental reactions to coming Out. In R. Dimitrova (Ed.), *Well-being of youth and emerging adults across cultures* (pp. 123–144). Springer. https://doi.org/10.1007/978-3-319-68363-8_9

Hayfield, N., Campbell, C., & Reed, E. (2018). Misrecognition and managing marginalisation: Bisexual people's experiences of bisexuality and relationships. *Psychology & Sexuality, 9*(3), 221–236. https://doi.org/10.1080/19419899.2018.1470106

Heatherington, L., & Lavner, J. A. (2008). Coming to terms with coming out: Review and recommendations for family systems-focused research. *Journal of Family Psychology, 22*(3), 329–343. https://doi.org/10.1037/0893-3200.22.3.329

Jaspal, R. (2020). Parental reactions to British South Asian young men who identify as gay. *Journal of GLBT Family Studies, 16*(4), 402–417. https://doi.org/10.1080/1550428X.2019.1684412

Jaspal, R. (2025a). A theoretical model for predicting outness in lesbian, gay and bisexual people: Minority stressors, social support, and identity processes. *Social Sciences, 14*(4), 207. https://doi.org/10.3390/socsci14040207

Jaspal, R. (2025b). Minority stressors, social connectedness and degree of outness in gay men: Data from two cross-sectional correlational studies in the United Kingdom. *Sexuality and Culture, 29*(3), 1318–1338. https://doi.org/10.1007/s12119-025-10325-4

Jaspal, R., & Cinnirella, M. (2010). Coping with potentially incompatible identities: Accounts of religious, ethnic, and sexual identities from British Pakistani men who identify as Muslim and gay. *British Journal of Social Psychology, 49*(4), 849–870. https://doi.org/10.1348/014466609X485025

Jaspal, R., & Siraj, A. (2011). Perceptions of 'coming out' among British Muslim gay men. *Psychology and Sexuality, 2*(3), 183–197. https://doi.org/10.1080/19419899.2010.526627

Johnston, L. B., & Jenkins, D. (2004). Coming out in mid-adulthood: Building a new identity. *Journal of Gay & Lesbian Social Services, 16*(2), 19–42. https://doi.org/10.1300/J041v16n02_02

Kashubeck-West, S., Whiteley, A. M., Vossenkemper, T., Robinson, C., & Deitz, C. (2017). Conflicting identities: Sexual minority, transgender, and gender nonconforming individuals navigating between religion and gender–sexual orientation identity. In K. A. DeBord, A. R. Fischer, K. J. Bieschke, & R. M. Perez (Eds.), *Handbook of sexual orientation and gender diversity in counseling and psychotherapy* (pp. 213–238). American Psychological Association. https://doi.org/10.1037/15959-009

Kim, H. M., Jeong, J. C., Appleby, P. R., Christensen, J. L., & Miller, L. C. (2021). Parental rejection after coming out: Detachment, shame, and the reparative power of romantic love. *International Journal of Communication, 15*, 3740–3759.

Kinsey, A. C., Pomeroy, W. B., & Martin, C. E. (1948). *Sexual behavior in the human male.* W. B. Saunders.

Landolt, M. A., Bartholomew, K., Saffrey, C., Oram, D., & Perlman, D. (2004). Gender nonconformity, childhood rejection, and adult attachment: A study of gay men. *Archives of Sexual Behavior, 33*(2), 117–128. https://doi.org/10.1023/b:aseb.0000014326.64934.50

McConnell, E. A., Birkett, M., & Mustanski, B. (2016). Families matter: Social support and mental health trajectories among lesbian, gay, bisexual, and transgender youth. *The Journal of Adolescent Health, 59*(6), 674–680. https://doi.org/10.1016/j.jadohealth.2016.07.026

McLean, K. (2007). Hiding in the closet? Bisexuals, coming out and the disclosure imperative. *Journal of Sociology, 43*(2), 151–166. https://doi.org/10.1177/1440783307076893

Meyer, I. H. (2003). Prejudice, social stress, and mental health in lesbian, gay, and bisexual populations: Conceptual issues and research evidence. *Psychological Bulletin, 129*(5), 674–697. https://doi.org/10.1037/0033-2909.129.5.674

Nordqvist, P., & Smart, C. (2014). Troubling the family: Coming out as lesbian and gay. *Families, Relationships and Societies, 3*(1), 97–112. https://doi.org/10.1332/204674313X667380

Orne, J. (2011). 'You will always have to "out" yourself': Reconsidering coming out through strategic outness. *Sexualities, 14*(6), 681–703. https://doi.org/10.1177/1363460711420462

Pachankis, J. E., Goldfried, M. R., & Ramrattan, M. E. (2008). Extension of the rejection sensitivity construct to the interpersonal functioning of gay men. *Journal of Consulting and Clinical Psychology, 76*(2), 306–317. https://doi.org/10.1037/0022-006X.76.2.306

Parra, L. A., Bell, T. S., Benibgui, M., Helm, J. L., & Hastings, P. D. (2018). The buffering effect of peer support on the links between family rejection and psychosocial adjustment in LGB emerging adults. *Journal of Social and Personal Relationships, 35*(6), 854–871. https://doi.org/10.1177/0265407517699713

Puckett, J. A., Woodward, E. N., Mereish, E. H., & Pantalone, D. W. (2015). Parental rejection following sexual orientation disclosure: Impact on internalized homophobia, social support, and mental health. *LGBT Health, 2*(3), 265–269. https://doi.org/10.1089/lgbt.2013.0024

Salerno, J. P., Gattamorta, K. A., & Williams, N. D. (2023). Impact of family rejection and racism on sexual and gender minority stress among LGBTQ young people of color during COVID-19. *Psychological Trauma Theory Research Practice and Policy, 15*(4), 637–647. https://doi.org/10.1037/tra0001254

Savin-Williams, R. C. (2001). *Mom, dad. I'm gay. How families negotiate coming out*. American Psychological Association. https://doi.org/10.1037/10437-000

Sumerau, J. E., Grollman, E. A., & Cragun, R. T. (2018). "Oh my God, I sound like a horrible person": Generic processes in the conditional acceptance of sexual and gender diversity. *Symbolic Interaction, 41*(1), 62–82. https://doi.org/10.1002/symb.326

Willoughby, B. L. B., & Doty, N. D. (2010). Brief cognitive behavioral family therapy following a child's coming out: A case report. *Cognitive and Behavioral Practice, 17*(1), 37–44. https://doi.org/10.1016/j.cbpra.2009.04.006

9

Psychological Violence: Microaggressions, Ghosting, and Gaslighting

Microaggressions

Microaggressions are subtle forms of everyday discrimination that may be intentional or unintentional, but communicate negative and hostile messages about one's minority identity, such as being lesbian, gay, or bisexual (LGB) (Nadal, 2023). As such, they can be viewed as identity hazards. Microaggressions are experienced in many different contexts, including in school settings, universities, the workplace, religious settings, the family, and, increasingly, in digital settings (Lomash et al., 2019; McInroy et al., 2024; Resnick & Galupo, 2019; Winberg et al., 2019). Microaggressions against LGB people are most commonly enacted by heterosexual people. However, there is also evidence that subgroups within the broader LGB community can enact microaggressions against one another. For instance, ethnic majority LGB people may direct racial microaggressions against LGB people of minority ethnic background (Jaspal, 2017), while gay and lesbian people may direct them against bisexual people (Matsick & Rubin, 2018). Power dynamics are said to be key to microaggressions (Tran et al., 2023).

R. Jaspal, *The Psychology of Coming Out*,
https://doi.org/10.1007/978-3-032-02599-9_9

There are now several quantitative scales that attempt to measure microaggressions. Wright and Wegner (2012) developed and validated the Homonegative Microaggressions Scale and found that it correlates negatively with self-esteem and positively with internalized homonegativity. Woodford et al. (2015) developed the LGBQ Microaggressions on College Campuses Scale which consists of two subscales focusing on interpersonal and environmental microaggressions. Swann et al. (2016) examined the psychometric properties of the Sexual Orientation Microaggression Inventory and, in addition to a general factor, identified four specific subfactors of microinsults (anti-gay attitudes), denial of homosexuality, microinvalidations (heterosexism), and microassaults (societal disapproval of homosexuality). Recognizing the uniqueness of microaggressions experienced within the family context, Sterzing and Gartner (2020) developed the LGBTQ Microaggressions and Microaffirmations in Families Scale which measures both subtle acts of discrimination as well as those that affirm the lesbian, gay, bisexual, transgender, queer, or questioning (LGBTQ) person's sexual identity. Both the microaggressions and microaffirmations subscales correlated with mental health variables and, additionally, the level of family religiosity was positively associated with microaggressions and negatively correlated with microaffirmations.

Experiences of microaggressions appear to be quite common in LGB people. McCabe et al. (2013) surveyed school psychologists regarding their observations of anti-LGBTQ bias and sexuality in their schools—16% reported observing bias and harassment once a month or more frequently and 43% reported hearing microaggressions, such as "that's so gay" (when referring to something negative) once a month or more frequently (sometimes from teachers themselves). School psychologists tended to respond to direct verbal insults but often ignored microaggressions that were not directed at individuals.

Qualitative focus group and individual interview research with young gay men in Mexico shows the pervasiveness of microaggressions in their lives, which can include interactions with family, friends, classmates at school, and which is associated with a range of negative emotions and coping strategies, such as concealment of sexuality (Mendoza-Pérez et al., 2024). Legge et al. (2018) analyzed the diary entries of 86 young bisexual people concerning their negative identity experiences. There was a strong focus upon microaggressions in their accounts with the majority reporting experiences of identity erasure and negative stereotyping of bisexual people.

LGB people of religious faith, in particular, commonly report experiences of microaggressions. Lomash et al. (2019) studied microaggressions in religious and spiritual contexts and found that microaggressions were used by religious people to indicate tolerance but not full acceptance of the LGB person's sexual identity. Moreover, they found that the notion of tolerance was mobilized to deny accusations of heterosexism and homonegativity (see also Cvetkovska et al., 2024). More generally, microaggressions were used to reinforce the social representation that LGB and religious identities are incompatible. In their qualitative interview study of Christian lesbian, gay, bisexual, and transgender (LGBT) teenagers and their parents, Sorrell et al. (2024a, b) found that they all experienced a variety of verbal, nonverbal, and environmental microaggressions. For instance, comments were made to suggest that they were not faithful members of the Church, that being LGBT was shameful, that being LGBT could be overcome, and that parents should limit their support for their LGBT children. In another study, Sorrell et al. (2024a, b) found that teens and their parents experienced a range of negative emotions, as well as religious doubt, disengagement, and disillusionment due to microaggressions.

Consistent with minority stress theory, empirical research unequivocally shows the negative effects of exposure to microaggressions for mental health. A study using diary methods found exposure to microaggressions to be associated with negative affect and even poor physical health outcomes in bisexual women (Smith et al., 2023). Furthermore, experiences of microaggressions were found to be associated with higher levels of depressive, anxious, and stress symptoms across four cross-sectional studies of Brazilian LGB people (Silva et al., 2025), as well as with post-traumatic stress symptoms (Robinson & Rubin, 2016). Systematic reviews of microaggressions against sexual minorities confirm their association with depression and anxiety but also with alcohol abuse, substance abuse, suicidal ideation, and suicide attempts, showing the broader mental health sequelae of experiencing microaggressions (DeSon & Andover, 2024; Marchi et al., 2024).

Some studies have also examined the mediating and moderating factors in the relationship between microaggressions exposure and poor mental health. In their study of 267 Dutch sexual minority youth, Kaufman et al. (2017) found that experiences of microaggressions were associated with depressive symptoms through the mediation of rumination. In other words, experiences of microaggressions may lead some sexual minority people to overthink what their experiences mean (possibly due to the inherent uncertainty associated with microaggressions) which in turn can lead to higher risk of depression. They did not find social support to have any buffering effects upon these relationships.

In their study of 186 LGBTQ emerging adults, Wike et al. (2023) found that the relationship between microaggressions and both anxiety and depression was moderated by thwarted belongingness. Only at high and moderate levels of thwarted belongingness were the relationships between microaggressions and depression and anxiety statistically significant. Similarly, in their study of 1292 Latino sexual and gender minority youth, Abreu et al. (2023) found that individuals exposed to intersectional microaggressions (due to their sexuality and ethnicity) and who also reported lower sexuality-specific parental support exhibited higher depressive symptoms. Furthermore, sexuality-specific parental support appeared only to be protective at lower, rather than higher, levels of intersectional microaggressions.

Abreu et al.'s (2023) study shows that particular subgroups of LGB people may face a multitude of microaggressions. In their systematic review of research into intersectional microaggressions among LGBTQ people of ethnic minority background in Canada, Sadika et al. (2020) found that individuals experienced microaggressions in their families and ethnic communities due to their sexuality and in sexuality-affirmative contexts due to their ethnicity, which could make it difficult to navigate their intersecting identities.

LGB people react to microaggressions in varied ways. In their qualitative study of 26 LGB people, Nadal et al. (2011) found a range of coping strategies deployed in response to microaggressions. At the cognitive level, some individuals felt empowered after experiencing microaggressions while others uncritically accepted that they would always be part of a LGB person's experience. At the behavioral level, some passively accepted the microaggressions and did nothing, while others actively confronted them. The choice of coping strategy depends on many factors, including the individual's personality, level of social support, and the social context. Moreover, microaggressions may be difficult to detect due to their subtlety, making it similarly difficult to enlist the support of others to challenge them collectively.

Gaslighting

Gaslighting refers to the act of manipulating another person into doubting himself or herself and thus questioning their own perceptions, reality, or even sanity, while denying that one is actually doing this (Akdeniz & Cıhan, 2024). One study found that 54.3% of cases of psychological aggression in relationships consisted of gaslighting, suggesting that this abusive behavior is relatively common (Kim et al., 2023). In their conceptual overview of gaslighting, Johnson et al. (2021) provide an overview of the various forms of gaslighting faced by members of minority groups, including LGB people, its psychological underpinnings, and the harms caused to victims of gaslighting.

There is remarkably little empirical research into experiences of gaslighting (Akdeniz & Cıhan, 2024) and even less research focusing specifically on LGB people. It does appear that exposure to gaslighting can have negative effects upon mental health. Gaslighting has been found to be associated with a diminished sense of self and the development of both self-doubt and mistrust of others (Hailes & Goodman, 2025). In their study of gaslighting in women, Güleç and Özbay (2024) found that exposure to gaslighting was directly and negatively associated with life satisfaction and that it was indirectly associated with life satisfaction through psychological resilience which appeared to operate as a protective factor. In their study of gaslighting in a sample with 287 heterosexual and 257 LGB people in the United Kingdom, Lopes and Jaspal (2025) found that gaslighting was positively associated with depression and that there were no statistically significant differences by sexual orientation, suggesting that LGB and heterosexual people are affected by gaslighting in a similar way (see also Jaspal & Lopes, 2025b).

The available evidence suggests that gaslighting constitutes an identity hazard. In an autoethnography, Wozolek (2018) refers to the pervasiveness of gaslighting against LGB young people as a social process in the school context. Li and Samp (2023) examined the individual and relational correlates of LGBTQ people's experiences of gaslighting and found that individuals with a more affirmative sexual identity and higher relational power (i.e., the level of power symmetry in the relationship) reported less gaslighting. Furthermore, gaslighting experiences were associated with poor mental and physical health outcomes, as well as more adverse relational satisfaction. Their study also provided interesting insight into the most common perpetrators of gaslighting from the perspective of LGBTQ people themselves. Fathers were most commonly identified as the main gaslighters, followed by mothers and male friends, and finally female friends.

In Li and Samp's (2023) study, common gaslighting experiences included devaluing and questioning the significance and validity of the LGB person's sexual identity, deliberately forgetting their coming out experience, and controlling conversations, as well as more subtle gaslighting tactics. Adverse communication behaviors, such as gaslighting, are also faced by LGB people in relation to other issues, such as their mental health and therapy following a traumatic childhood experience, such as childhood sexual abuse (Dorri et al., 2024). A cross-sectional survey study examined the prevalence of gaslighting experiences in LGBTQ people specifically in medical contexts and found that almost half of all LGBTQ respondents reported gaslighting which was significantly higher than among heterosexual people. They also reported less trust in healthcare institutions and in health providers which echoes the findings of studies of LGB people in other empirical contexts (e.g., Jolley & Jaspal, 2020).

Ghosting

Ghosting refers to the act of ending a relationship with somebody suddenly by ceasing all communication with them and usually occurs within digital settings, such as on social media or instant messaging (Freedman et al., 2022). Ghosting appears to be very common—a recent study of undergraduate students in the United States found that more than half of recent breakups involved ghosting (Collins et al., 2023). Similarly, in their study of victimization experiences in 544 men and women in the United Kingdom (Jaspal & Lopes, 2025a), 60% of the sample reported ever having experienced ghosting from a dating partner. Ghosting has been observed in a wide range of relationship types. People generally report greater ease in ghosting friends and acquaintances with whom they are not romantically involved compared to those with whom they are romantically involved (e.g., Leckfor et al., 2023).

Much research into ghosting focuses on the motives for enacting ghosting, that is, on the psychology of perpetrators. Some studies provide insight into the situational factors that increase the likelihood of perpetrating this type of behavior—for instance, Wu and Bamishigbin (2023) note that the desire to avoid confrontation is a key factor and that the perpetrator often recognizes the harm caused (see also Collins et al., 2023). Freedman et al. (2022) have shown that safety concerns may make women more likely to ghost men, especially when the male target is perceived as being dangerous.

The consequences of ghosting for mental health are well documented and there is evidence that exposure to this particular behavior is more harmful to mental health than rejection *per se* (Pancani et al., 2022). People who experience ghosting report feeling sad and distressed (Pancani et al., 2021). They may experience threats to fundamental psychological needs, such as self-esteem, belonging, meaning, and self-efficacy (Freedman et al., 2024; Konings et al., 2023; Pancani et al., 2022), as well as anxiety (Forrai et al., 2023) and heightened uncertainty (LeFebvre et al., 2019). The uncertainty inherent to ghosting is perhaps what makes this behavior so insidious. In a similar vein, Lopes and Jaspal (2025) found that exposure to ghosting in their heterosexual and LGB samples was associated with increased paranoid ideation and that there were no statistically significant differences by sexual orientation (see also Jaspal & Lopes, 2025b). When ghosting is used in response to coming out, it can be viewed as an identity hazard for LGB people.

Ghosting has generally been examined in social media contexts. Studies of social media usage show that younger people use social media more intensively than older people (Astleitner et al., 2023) and that social media "unfollowing" and "unfriending," that is, ceasing connections on social networking platforms, such as Instagram or Facebook, is a key means of ghosting (Collins et al., 2023). Thus, younger adults may be especially vulnerable to ghosting than older adults. Navarro et al. (2020) did not find significant differences in ghosting by gender, sexual orientation, age, or current relationship status. There is limited empirical insight into ghosting experiences in LGB people (though see Lopes & Jaspal, 2025; Navarro et al., 2020), and none that examines ghosting from significant others following a coming out experience.

Written Accounts from Lesbian, Gay, and Bisexual People

In this section, the following three themes arising from the thematic analysis of LGB people's written accounts are described: (1) microaggressions; (2) ghosting; and (3) gaslighting.

Microaggressions

Individuals described experiencing a wide range of microaggressions from people to whom they came out:

> Though my college best friend did not condemn me, we have drifted farther apart since I told him about my sexuality. I do not talk to him as often on the phone, and I have a lesser opinion of some of his views (e.g., he is a Christian and claims to be okay with homosexuality only via a rather

offensive "hate the sin not the sinner" mentality). Distance from my best friend is a negative change resulting from my coming out.

The respondent reported that they were not explicitly condemned by their best friend but that they felt that their relationship with them changed negatively after they came out. The Christian notion of "hate the sin, not the sinner," which underpinned the negative change in their relationship, exemplifies the microaggressions faced by some LGB people when they come out. There was no suggestion that they were disliked but an important element of identity (i.e., their sexuality) was subtly denigrated.

Several respondents reported being excluded from events and gatherings which they attributed to homonegativity:

> Went to an all boys school and collectively I was kept at arm's length once I came out. It was not a nice feeling for the remainder of school. No-one was outright nasty but I would not go out of my way to speak to anyone I went to school with nowadays.

> No longer invited out with other heterosexual friends. This has never been made explicit but it is quite obvious that this is the case.

> I wasn't invited to parties anymore and when I raised this my friends basically said they thought I wouldn't enjoy myself because there were no other gay people there. Basically I was too gay for their parties after coming out.

As highlighted in the extracts, emotional distance was construed in terms of being "kept at arm's length" rather than "outright nasty" and as "no longer [being] invited out" rather than "explicit." Nevertheless, individuals knew instinctively that they were being shunned and, in some cases, experienced prolonged psychological distress: "it was not a nice feeling for the remainder of school." According to one participant's account, their friend made the (erroneous) assumption that they would not enjoy themselves "because there were no other gay people there," essentially assuming that gay people only enjoy themselves in the presence of other gay people. Comments of this kind draw unwanted attention to individuals' sexuality even in contexts in which this is deemed to be irrelevant or in which LGB people themselves do not wish for this to be relevant.

Participants in the sample described other passive forms of prejudice manifested in terms of negative changes that occurred in their relationships with others:

> I feel like I am constantly having to prove to them that I am "normal." I feel our relationship shifted after I came out to them where we ironically can't be as free around each other.
>
> My mother was more attentive toward me. I couldn't have some sort of life outside of my home. She was just worried someone will hurt me all because I'm gay.
>
> Couldn't have boys stay over after coming out to my mum.
>
> After that, there was a lot of suspicion about every male friend I had as in "oh you must be having sex with them" so my parents basically assumed I was sex-mad and made this known to me very clearly.

One respondent reported feeling the necessity to "prove" that they were "normal" after coming out. This could be attributed to the sudden changes in their relationships with others after they came out to them. In short, they were not explicitly told that they were abnormal but were made to feel as such because they were treated differently: "we ironically can't be as free around each other."

Furthermore, participants' written statements highlight novel restrictions imposed on them following their coming out experience. One individual felt scrutinized by their mother who no longer allowed them to "have some sort of life outside of [their] home" while another participant's mother reportedly did not allow him to have male friends staying over. Significant others drew unwanted negative attention to coming-out individuals' sexuality. In the case of one respondent, it was implied that his sexuality made him vulnerable to stigma, denigration, and attacks from others, and that being gay perhaps "weakened" him somewhat. Incidentally, this assumption was inconsistent with how the individual himself felt about his sexuality. In the case of others, it was implied that they were sexually promiscuous and attracted to *all* other individuals of the same sex simply because they were LGB. Same-sex friendships were sometimes mistaken for possible sexual relationships. In all four accounts above, coming out did not precipitate an overtly prejudicial response but it did generate negative changes that signaled significant others' negative appraisal of their sexual identity. These were subtle but palpable negative reactions from valued others.

Some respondents described their significant others' attempts to explain their negative reactions and behaviors after coming out. In several cases, it was suggested that they reacted negatively because of fears and concerns about individuals' current or future wellbeing because they were LGB:

> When I came out to my family, my mother didn't believe me, relabeled my sexuality, insisted she didn't care who I dated and essentially didn't want to know about it. I was quite insecure in my identity so this hurt me a lot. When I asked her recently about how she felt when I first came out to her, she said she was disappointed and frightened because she didn't want me to face discrimination or hardship. I think that explains why she reacted the way that she did.

In several accounts, individuals' significant others claimed to be accepting or indifferent but their behavior suggested that they in fact construed their offspring's sexuality negatively. The participant's mother expressed disbelief and refused to recognize their sexual identity by "relabeling" it. As noted by several respondents, microaggressions of this kind were psychologically distressing and could also contribute to feelings of identity doubt. Yet, the explanation given to the participant by their mother could also be viewed in terms of a microaggression. Their mother assumed and implied that their sexuality would expose them to "discrimination or hardship," which was inconsistent with the individual's own construal of their sexual identity. Moreover, their sexuality was said to constitute a source of disappointment and fear for their mother.

> When I came out to a particular person, though they came to terms with it relatively quickly and accepted who I was, they felt that more could have been done to prevent it. They also felt pity and concern that I wouldn't have a traditional family/life as they did rearing children and being a

> parent. I think they are needlessly worrying about me when they shouldn't be as I am an adult capable of making my own decision.

> They started to get involved in my business and giving me unwanted advice and telling me what to do. They wanted to help but were not always giving positive advice.

One participant's significant other "felt that more could have been done to prevent it" while "worrying" and expressing "pity and concern." This reaction constitutes a microaggression because, in spite of the superficial acceptance offered by the individual's significant others, they suggested that the individual's sexuality was changeable and that it would have been preferable for them to be heterosexual. Although they did not blame or target the coming-out individual directly, they reportedly felt inadequate because they had been unable to "prevent" their homosexuality. Another respondent reported unwanted advice and invasion of their privacy as well as forms of coercion from their significant others because they were deemed to need help due to their sexual orientation. All this indicated to coming-out individuals that their sexuality was problematic, flawed, and worthy of shame. When LGB people come out to their significant others, they are generally seeking validation, approval, and acceptance of their sexual identity. Yet, they sometimes encounter negative emotional reactions.

These accounts converge in showing the apparent acceptance but more subtle microaggressions that some coming-out LGB individuals face. They were manifested primarily in expressions of pity and concern, as well as the assumption that, because they were coming out as LGB, individuals automatically faced vulnerability and should therefore be protected. As one participant's account demonstrated, some LGB people are made to feel vulnerable and incapable of taking their own decisions about their lives, with potential repercussions for feelings of self-efficacy. Furthermore, it was noted that the advice and guidance they received were not positive or consistent with the identities that they wished to construct.

Some participants reported facing an undesirable foregrounding of their sexuality upon coming out:

> Being treated as if I was a new person and in a way that made the focus of my interactions with them solely focus on being queer.
>
> I sometimes feel like they expect me to act in a certain way, like they want me to live up to a stereotype that they have of what they think being gay means.
>
> I remember coming out to someone in middle school, and there seemed to be a change in how they perceived my desires. For example, when I told them I was gay, as if suddenly, it seemed like the only thing I wanted was something up my ass.

As highlighted in Chap. 6, the continuation of interpersonal relationships was a key characteristic of positive coming out experiences. Coming-out individuals do not necessarily wish for their sexuality to become a dominant feature of their identity when they come out. Yet, this occurred for some. As one participant noted, their sexuality "became the focus of my interactions with them" while another perceived a social expectation for them to "act in a certain way." Both the pervasive foregrounding of their sexuality and the imposition of a stereotype that was inconsistent with their identity could engender threats to continuity, as indicated by one respondent who reported being treated as "a new person." Some observed changes in how they were subsequently perceived by others. In this case, there was an additional layer of complexity: the reduction of their sexuality to sex. Indeed, this was a recurrent type of microaggression described by participants in the sample:

> A male friend in particular thought it was an invitation to discuss my sexual activity and whether or not this meant my partner and I were open to threesomes. More generally I'm acutely aware of how fetishized bi women are.
>
> They started treating me differently. They acted as if I was a predator just because I am attracted to the same sex.
>
> My cousins asked me some very intimate questions about my bisexuality like if I was capable of being faithful to my girlfriend because I also like guys and they were constantly implying that I'm sex-starved and just want sex, be it with guys or girls. It is a fetishization of us bisexuals.

Not only was sexuality undesirably rendered salient when some people came out as LGB but also sexualized by others. Respondents felt “fetishized” by remarks about their sexuality and lamented that this level of intrusiveness was deemed acceptable when they came out as LGB. Incidentally, such intrusiveness was observed by other participants who noted that uncomfortable questions were asked about their sex lives:

> Get asked lots of questions that I don’t believe would be asked of heterosexual people such as “how do you have sex?”
>
> My brother makes jokes that my other siblings laugh at like mentioning “scissors” when referring to me as in I like “scissoring other girls.”

One respondent felt that, because they had same-sex attractions, they were treated as “a predator.” Some were teased about sexual practices stereotypically associated with their sexual orientation group. Another respondent believed that they were snubbed by their friend—the assumption was made that, because they were LGB, they were attracted to their (male) friend. Similarly, one individual noted that they were automatically assumed to be attracted to all other homosexual men:

> Think that just because I’m homosexual I’m automatically attracted to someone else who is also homosexual.
>
> My cousin made this really ridiculous comment when I came out to him basically that “oh just so you know, I like girls, not guys” and I was thinking “even if you were the last guy on the planet I would vomit on you rather than get with you” but still it felt like an attack.
>
> Best friend’s response was to remind me that he’s straight as if I was into him.

These experiences share a common feature—the sexualization of the coming-out individual’s sexual identity which is foregrounded over and above all other identity elements. They were perceived as subtle attacks on identity and, as such, can be regarded as microaggressions.

Ghosting

Respondents described being ghosted by significant others when they came out to them. More specifically, they noted that the relationship was not clearly and definitively terminated, nor was disapproval explicitly communicated to them. Rather, communication was abruptly severed and they felt ignored by people that mattered to them:

> My best friend literally stopped replying to my texts and just acted like I was invisible. He blocked me on social media and everything. He later apologized and we got over it but at the time it was horrible.

As the participant noted, ghosting was frequently enacted in online settings with several individuals noting that they stopped receiving responses to their text messages, often from people with whom they had previously had regular contact (in this case, their best friend). Furthermore, a common ghosting technique was being "blocked" or "unfollowed" on social media. In many cases, there was ambiguity because they were not explicitly told that they were being blocked but rather could no longer locate others' profiles on social media or suddenly realized that they had fewer followers. Some attributed this to their coming out. Several individuals provided some insight into how ghosting made them feel. The participant cited above reported feeling "invisible" and described the experience at the time as horrible, although the relationship was eventually repaired.

Other manifestations of ghosting were also reported. For instance, some described being subtly ignored or sidelined by friends who had previously involved them in collective activities:

> I stopped getting invited to things and my male friends kept me at arm's length. I felt like I had some contagious disease or something. Actually they just didn't want people thinking they were gay.

> My friends would plan stuff and not invite me. If I asked about it on socials, they'd see the message but not reply and ignore me, basically ignore me. I just stopped existing for them so I had to rethink my options and I just distanced myself from them and made more accepting friends.

In some cases, individuals reported not being invited to events and gatherings to which they previously would have been invited and, in others, they recalled being ignored on social media when they attempted to contact friends. This contributed to feelings of invisibility—indeed, one participant felt that they "stopped existing for them" and another felt like he "had some contagious disease or something." This exemplifies the stigma that underpinned the ghosting experiences to which they were exposed. Respondents attempted to attribute meaning to their experiences of ghosting and deduced that their friends did not wish to be associated with them due to their sexual identity.

Some participants' accounts provided insight into their strategies for managing and coping with these threatening experiences—in some cases, they reached the conclusion that their friends no longer wished to continue the friendship due to their coming out. Some sought to replace these friendships with others that were more accommodating of their sexuality.

Ghosting has generally been reported in the context of romantic relationships and friendships (Lopes & Jaspal, 2025). However, participants' written accounts also showed that this behavior was relatively common among their family members following a negative coming out experience:

> My relationship with my mother took a downward spiral and things got very messy. She ignored my texts and basically the let's-make-conversation texts that don't mean much. I remember going home and just thinking "what kind of atmosphere am I walking into, the type you can cut with a knife?" I felt a lot of fear after coming out.

As in the previous examples of ghosting from friends, here the participant reported the sudden change in their relationship with their mother after coming out. They had previously exchanged text messages but, when they came out, their mother stopped responding to them. The participant continued to live with their mother but reported being ignored—primarily in text messages—which, for them, evidenced a breakdown in their relationship. This in turn created a stressful situation in the home environment since they worried about the negative atmosphere that would exist at home and whether the distance observed in text messages would be similarly observable in in-person interactions with their mother. Others reported similar ghosting experiences from their family members:

> After I came out to my parents the communication just stopped really. I sent a WhatsApp to my mum, she read it straightaway but would not reply and then I talked to my sister and she was replying to her but ignoring me. She thought less of me because I'm a lesbian.

In this particular case, the respondent noted that her parents stopped communicating with her via text message after she came out. She attributed this to her coming out experience because her mother reportedly continued to communicate with her sister but not with her. As in other accounts of ghosting, this signaled exclusion and rejection, as well as her parents' disapproval of her sexuality: "she thought less of me because I'm a lesbian." Individuals' accounts showed that ghosting could also extend beyond their immediate family members to others in their social circles:

> I came out to my folks during my year abroad in Spain. I told them and they seemed OK but then I got there and they ignored my calls, texts, and emails. I called my aunt and she was very superficial and then radio-silence after that. It was the worst period of my life. I felt really nervous and didn't know what was going to happen. And I felt very unloved.

LGB people come out in many different ways and, given that the prospect of coming out can be stressful, some choose to come out when they are no longer living with their parents. This can provide some psychological safety in relation to a potentially stress-inducing experience. The participant decided to come out to their parents while abroad but expected to retain contact with their parents. However, they were ghosted: "they ignored my calls, texts and emails." Ghosting in this way can deprive coming-out individuals of the ability to engage with their significant others about their sexual identity, which is important for moving toward interpersonal understanding and reconciliation. The participant reported initially being ghosted by their parents and subsequently by their aunt whom they attempted to contact. Like others who reported experiences of ghosting, this participant felt nervous due to the uncertainty about the status of their relationships. They did not actually know what this behavior signified. Furthermore, they reported feeling "unloved" and even deemed this "the worst period of my life." Clearly, these experiences were psychologically impactful and, in some cases, made individuals regret having come out in the first place.

Gaslighting

One of the most insidious adverse reactions that participants reported was that of gaslighting from significant others when they came out as LGB. They were made to doubt the reality of their sexuality or to feel that they had let down their significant others. In the latter case, coming-out individuals were vilified rather than supported. It is important to note the psychological significance of coming out for many LGB people for whom this tends to be a key milestone in their sexual identity development. Yet, several participants reported that they did not receive support but denigration due to purported dishonesty, which constituted a form of gaslighting:

> My friend at the time no longer speaks to me due to me coming out. They made me coming out about themselves, like I was keeping a secret from them, rather than being happy for me for living my truth. We no longer speak.
>
> After coming out to a close friend of mine of several years they expressed disgust and immediately claimed I'd been lying and deceiving them. They ceased contact with me and on occasion would call me slurs and threaten to hurt me if I went near them because they believed I was trying to hide my identity in order to take advantage of them.

In neither case is homonegativity particularly overt. Rather, it is expressed by constructing the coming-out person as dishonest and Machiavellian. One respondent was treated as if they were "keeping a secret from them" and another as someone "trying to hide" their (sexual) identity with an ulterior motive. Rather than attempting to understand the challenges associated with sexual identity development in a heteronormative society in which many face homonegativity, some participants' significant others reprimanded them for hiding their sexuality. It is easy to see how this response could affect people's self-esteem, not only due to the stigma appended to their sexuality but also to their decision not to come out sooner. This should also be viewed against the backdrop of dominant social representations of coming out discussed in Chap. 1.

Although some individuals felt that their sexual identity was initially accepted by significant others when they came out to them, they felt that this information was later "weaponized" or held against them:

> When I first came out to my mother, she was supportive and loving and wonderful. However, one week later, we got into an argument about something completely unrelated and she called me a homophobic slur. She'd never done this before, and I think she knew it hurt me quite deeply. Since then, there has been a bit of a barrier between myself and her.

The fact that the individual was denigrated due to their sexual identity following the apparently accommodating response from their mother suggested that their sexual identity was not really accepted. It was retained in the arsenal of possible psychological weapons to be used in arguments and deployed as such, which reportedly created "a barrier" between them in their relationship.

> After telling my parents, they both became really sympathetic and started telling me I was confused and that my uncle had gone through this but he turned out OK. They were making me feel like I had gone mad, just treating me like a confused sick person who would recover with the right treatment.

> My mum told me everything would be fine if I just got myself a girlfriend and that I would get over it eventually. I felt like I was being abused but with the nicest words. It was totally an attack on my persona.

Respondents' accounts of their negative coming out experiences suggest that gaslighting can consist of significant others' attempts to cause confusion by providing "evidence" that the coming-out individual is mistaken about their sexuality. For instance, one individual reported that their significant others had cited an uncle who "had gone through this" but who "turned out OK." This anecdote was intended to show that it is possible to change one's sexual orientation. When individuals come out as LGB, they are essentially sharing an important aspect of their identity. They are telling others who they are. Gaslighting constitutes a means of causing the individual to doubt this. In the extract above, the respondent describes his mother's attempt to provide a "solution," that is, for him to establish a heterosexual relationship which would reportedly enable him to "get over it eventually."

The psychological consequences of gaslighting were powerfully described in the corpus of written accounts. One individual felt that their sanity was doubted as they were treated "like a confused sick person" while others themselves appeared to be confused by the behavior that they experienced. Another respondent described their gaslighting experience as an "attack on my persona," highlighting the threat to identity. They felt that they were "being abused" though in a subtle manner that was perhaps difficult to call out as abuse.

Some respondents recognized the reaction from significant others to their coming out as gaslighting and described it as such:

> My parents were both gaslighting me from the first conversation. They said it was just hormones getting the better of me. They told me what they wanted to believe and wanted me to believe it but didn't care about my sanity in the process.

> My mum said "you are crying out for help" and "we are listening to you now" as if me coming out to them was some kind of protest. I was telling them who I was. It was the most invalidating gaslighting experience ever.

As noted earlier, many specific strategies were used by significant others to invalidate the coming-out individual's sexual identity. As seen in the extracts above, the coming-out individual's sexuality was attributed to "hormones" and to "protest," suggesting that this was a phase that could be overcome. Individuals were aware that these statements reflected what their significant others wished to believe because the reality of being LGB was unacceptable to them. These gaslighting experiences were psychologically harmful—respondents described the impact on their mental wellbeing ("my sanity") and their sense of identity: "it was the most invalidating gaslighting experience ever."

Some participants felt that they were manipulated by their significant others when coming out:

> When I came out to my father he was very supportive at first but then my brother showed me some messages where he was saying he should take me out to meet girls. I confronted him days later and he talked to me like I was stupid saying I was misunderstanding him. He got angry with me and I felt like I was in the wrong.

Gaslighting could occur because coming-out individuals were under the impression that their significant others accepted them and that they had their best interests at heart. One respondent recounted being led to believe that his father was supportive of his sexual identity but later learning that he had conspired with his brother to attempt to change his sexual orientation. The gaslighting reportedly continued when he confronted his father about this incident. He was made to feel "stupid" and that he "was in the wrong" despite knowing that it was his father who had in fact deceived him. In other words, the experience led him to doubt his reality. Similarly, others described the psychological violence perpetrated by significant others:

> They told me I was being a bit extreme with my reaction when I told them I'm gay and it felt like they were portraying themselves as the victim and me as the aggressor when I was sharing the most intimate thing about me.

As indicated by the respondent in their account, they were castigated by a significant other when they came out. More specifically, they were accused of reacting in an extreme manner and felt as if they were being treated as "the aggressor" in the situation. Conversely, they believed that their significant others portrayed themselves as "the victim." This reaction had at least two effects: on the one hand, it shifted the focus from the individual sharing an intimate aspect of their identity to the (negative) effect upon others and, on the other hand, it constructed the individual's coming out as an attack against others. This type of gaslighting evoked feelings of guilt.

Interview Accounts from Lesbian, Gay, and Bisexual People

In this section, the following three themes arising from the thematic analysis of participants' interview accounts are described: (1) microaggressions, self-esteem, and silence; (2) ghosting, uncertainty, and identity doubt; and (3) gaslighting, identity doubt, and (re)construal.

Microaggressions, Self-Esteem, and Silence

Interviewees described some of the microaggressions that they encountered upon coming out to significant others. Their accounts highlighted both the effects of exposure to microaggressions for their psychological wellbeing and the difficulties in addressing these microaggressions due to their subtlety:

> My dad was saying that bisexual people have it hard in life because they have trouble making their mind up but he was saying it like sympathetically and I was thinking that I don't really want their sympathy. It's more their love and understanding I want. I reckon if they had just been quiet and said nothing but transmitted positive energy, yes, it would have been a good coming out experience. But I just felt really bad about my sexuality and did for a long time because that idea of being bi and messed up just stuck in my head for a long time, making me think it was true. (James, bisexual man)

Several interviewees indicated that they had not been overtly stigmatized but rather that responses to coming out from significant others sometimes indicated that their sexuality was problematic. Indeed, James' father suggested that "bisexual people have it hard in life" and attributed this to bisexual people's indecisiveness. In this particular case, the tone of the comment was allegedly positive and "sympathetic" and thus could not be easily challenged. His father presented himself as a well-wisher concerned about his son's wellbeing. However, the underlying meaning was negative—a stigmatizing generalization was made about bisexuals and was similarly applied to James. James reported that the desired response would have been one of "love and understanding" but that the stigmatizing response he actually received challenged his sense of self-esteem: "I just felt really bad about my sexuality and did for a long time."

Microaggressions of this kind from people who really mattered appeared to be internalized by some coming-out individuals with lasting effects on their sense of identity: "the idea of being bi and messed up just stuck in my head for a long time, making me think it was true." Microaggressions can be difficult to detect and thus challenge. All interviewees recounted at least one story of an adverse reaction to their coming out, where their interlocutor responded in an overtly stigmatizing manner. Many also described more subtle forms of stigma:

> I can't put my finger on it because it wasn't a really, really bad reaction as in tantrums. There was just that, reading between the lines, it was like they really didn't like what they were hearing so they said few things that like if I repeat to you now you'll be like "oh that's not so bad" but it felt like a knife. The sort of thing like "I don't want you to get mixed up with the wrong crowd" or "I don't want you to get AIDS" and then crying but telling me they love me in the same breath. (Joe, gay man)

The microaggressions highlighted in Joe's account draw upon the negative social representations that associate gay men with illicit activity (e.g., promiscuity, drug use) and with HIV/AIDS (Jaspal & Nerlich, 2017). Joe's account showed how stigma can be presented as concern for the coming-out individual's wellbeing and accompanied by reassurance of love and sympathy. Joe himself interpreted this as evidence that "they really didn't like what they were hearing," which in turn caused him distress: "it felt like a knife." The significance of the threat to self-esteem could be attributed to the significance of the people creating the threat—they mattered to him.

> I actually cared more what my aunt thought about me because she was my everything. When I told her she said she was sorry for failing me in my upbringing and that was really painful because I just felt a massive shame and I knew I had let her down then and it just made me feel a lesser person, someone not really worthy of respect. I mean, I didn't really respect myself for months after that. (Jill, lesbian woman)

A common microaggression described by interviewees concerned the suggestion that their caregiver had "failed" them in some way which was purported to be the cause of their sexual orientation. As in the previous examples of microaggressions, the caregiver was reportedly apologetic, which framed their approach as one of care and concern. Jill described the psychological impact of this microaggression. It was described as "really painful" and as inducing shame and low self-esteem: "a lesser person, someone not really worthy of respect." As in other cases of microaggressions, this one had lasting effects on Jill who reported low self-esteem for a prolonged period of time. Crucially, this was so impactful because her caregiver was somebody that mattered. Moreover, a stigmatizing response that is framed as sympathy can be difficult to contest and perhaps more distressing than one that is more overt. Indeed, some interviewees reported finding it difficult to seek support in relation to the microaggressions that they faced from significant others upon coming out to them:

> Nobody really understands me when I try to get some support with my feelings about coming out [to other Christians]. I tell friends about the way my folks made me feel but nobody really gets it and that makes me feel really helpless, as in a bit invisible. I have started questioning if I'm just overreacting but I'm not really. It was all in their tone and in the things they were saying, like implying if you get me. This is for real but I did go through that phrase of doubt because of it. (Sally, lesbian woman)

A key characteristic of microaggressions is their subtlety which can make it difficult to explain them to others and enlist their support. Indeed, Sally noted that she did not feel understood when she attempted to explain these experiences to others and that her friends did not "really get it," generating feelings of helplessness and invisibility. It is easy to see how microaggressions could undermine not only self-esteem but also feelings of self-efficacy. Yet, exposure to microaggressions can have more insidious effects. As noted by Sally, she began to question her own judgment in response to others' incomprehension and entered a phase of doubt. Others similarly noted their doubts about their own judgment when exposed to microaggressions from significant others:

> I think the problem for me is I've never really been able to tell my friends how much their microaggressions hurt me at the time because they are microaggressions and so everything I say is basically justified or I'm the one who overreacted or misunderstood. Basically it's gaslighting. That is what happens when I try talking about it and it is frustrating. I can't really reconcile and we can't put this to bed because we can't talk about it honestly. (Jamie, bisexual woman)

As noted in Chap. 6, effective communication in the aftermath of coming out is important to LGB people even when the initial coming out experience is not entirely positive. Yet, microaggressions appeared to constitute a barrier to effective communication for some interviewees who felt unable to challenge these experiences or even to communicate how they made them feel. Similarly, Jamie indicated that she and her significant others had been unable to resolve the problems that underpinned their relationship. In her words, "we can't put this to bed because we can't talk about it honestly." Some were told, or made to feel, that they were "overreacting" and thus felt silenced:

> There was silence about all the jabs against me. To be honest, I don't think they were all intentional, like they were trying to hurt my feelings but they didn't get some of the words they were using like "oh I thought you were normal" as in using "normal" for "straight" but my point being I couldn't really tell them how much it was affecting my wellbeing. It was making me feel like shit but it was so tough to explain and they wouldn't have got it and they wouldn't have seen the damage to my mindset. I just felt really low, like really down, like I was being gaslit and there was nothing I could do about it, helpless really. (Janet, lesbian woman)

The social representation of abnormality in relation to homosexuality was mobilized in acts of microaggressions, whereby heterosexuality was constructed as "normal" and, thus, by implication homosexuality was constructed as "abnormal." Janet did not believe that this was necessarily malicious in intent but, like many others, felt gaslighted, silenced, and thus unable to challenge the behavior. Her account suggested that effective communication about these experiences and how they were making her feel could have enabled her to resolve them with her significant others, thereby potentially improving or restoring their relationship. However, this was not possible. Consequently, these microaggressions took their toll on her identity. Indeed, in Janet's account, the effects for self-esteem were evident: "it was making me feel like shit… the damage to my mindset…. I just felt really low, like really down." Moreover, the situation was described as "so tough" because of her helplessness, suggesting that her sense of self-efficacy was also undermined.

Ghosting, Uncertainty, and Identity Doubt

Several interviewees noted that ghosting from significant others upon coming out generated feelings of uncertainty and identity doubt:

> One of the most stressful situations for me was the knowing-but-not-knowing aspect of it all. They were just really off with me all the time and not replying to me when I texted or called but then the dinner would be on the table and it was all just really horrible. I was just made to feel like someone who had let them and the family down but still they were doing their duty of giving me food. As in "we love you but we don't like you." It really impacted on the feeling I had toward myself for a long time. (Ali, gay man)

As Ali noted, his parents' behavior toward him changed suddenly when he came out to them and he felt that he received mixed messages from them. On the one hand, they continued to provide for him (e.g., food and accommodation) but, on the other hand, they ceased to respond to his calls and messages. Their reaction was indicative of ghosting. Several interviewees in the sample described the uncertainty that this induced—they were unable to predict the future and, particularly, how their relationship with significant others might evolve. Yet, they attempted to ascribe meaning to these experiences. Ali interpreted this inconsistent behavior as evidence that his parents continued to love him and to comply with their perceived responsibility toward him as his parents but that they no longer "liked" him because of his sexuality. He noted the adverse impact that it had on his self-esteem, in particular. It was perhaps the inconsistency of his parents' behavior that led him to question his own identity—they continued to meet his material needs but no longer connected with him on an emotional level and clearly communicated to him their disapproval of his sexual identity.

Experiences of ghosting from friends and acquaintances were far more common in the participant sample:

> I stopped getting invited to stuff and knew that I'd been blocked by a couple of people but then in the corridors at university there was still the small talk and the questions about my weekend but I could see the fakeness of it all. Our conversations had become really superficial after I came out and it wasn't like before. I was being ghosted online by them because it was really like I didn't exist anymore but they made an effort in person. It was really horrible at the time because even I started asking myself if I was a terrible person, like a leper or something for them to treat me like this and in this day and age. (Bill, gay man)

For some interviewees, moving away from the family home was a positive step that allowed them and their significant others some time to recalibrate following their coming out experience. They had held positive expectations about the impact that going into novel spaces (e.g., university, as in the case of Bill) would have on their identity and wellbeing. Yet, their actual experiences did not always match expectations. For instance, Bill described being ghosted by university friends whom he had expected to be accepting of his sexual identity when he came out to them. The ghosting experiences consisted of negative changes in their level of intimacy ("our conversations had become really superficial"), being excluded from invitations and social gatherings ("I stopped getting invited to stuff"), and, in some cases, relations being severed in online settings ("I'd been blocked by a couple of people").

Bill perceived mixed messages from his university friends who, on the one hand, ghosted him but, in face-to-face contexts, appeared to engage with him, albeit superficially. The more significant observation from his account is the way these experiences of ghosting from people whom he had trusted made him feel about his own identity. He began to experience doubts about his identity, most notably his self-esteem: "I started asking myself if I was a terrible person, like a leper or something." It is easy to see how the conflict between his expectation of acceptance and his lived experience of ghosting may also challenge his sense of continuity. Indeed, continuity was challenged in other reported experiences of ghosting:

> My so-called best friend—let's call him that because that's what he was to me then at that point—well, he just cut all contact with me and didn't say why but putting two and two together, it was basically because I had come out as gay and he couldn't hack it. He just couldn't handle it and, yeah, I was really in shock about that. He never told me face-to-face that we weren't friends so I guess I lived with the hope that he'd come round and did live with that kind of hope so I tried several times but nothing came of it. That hope of getting back our friendship stayed though I gave up and moved on. (Aaron, gay man)

Aaron reported the breakdown of his relationship with his best friend after coming out to him. Crucially, his friend reportedly severed all contact with him without providing an explanation or even clarifying that the friendship had ended. This led to feelings of uncertainty about the status of the friendship although Aaron attributed this to his coming out. This was clearly challenging for continuity because of the sudden negative change in a valued relationship. Furthermore, the uncertainty that characterized this experience perhaps rendered it more threatening for identity: "he never told me face-to-face we weren't friends." Aaron attempted to recuperate the friendship, but to no avail, and thus resigned himself to the reality that the friendship was indeed over: "that hope of getting back our friendship stayed though I gave up and moved on."

Uncertainty is central to ghosting and can itself introduce uncertainty in identity:

> I think the hardest thing for me about having all ties cut with me after coming out was just the not knowing. The fact that I didn't know is we were on or off. If my mate still wanted to be my mate or if we could work through this and if he could accept me or not. It just became hard to have a conversation to straighten things out because he just vanished online and I couldn't get hold of him. Yeah so for me it was just the not knowing and the guessing game and the eggshells. It affected me a lot at the time and to be honest thinking about it still does too. I started to like believe all sorts about the situation, myself. (Michael, gay man)

For interviewees who reported experiencing ghosting, the most challenging aspect of the experience was the uncertainty inherent to it: "the not knowing and the guessing game." Like many others, Michael indicated that his friend "just vanished online" without explanation when he came out as gay. Several interviewees who experienced ghosting attempted unsuccessfully to repair the relationship. They were not given the opportunity to discuss the matter following the original coming out experience. As Michael noted, this experience had a profoundly negative impact upon his psychological wellbeing and reportedly still did. He alluded to the doubts he consequently experienced in relation to his own identity: "I started to like believe all sorts about the situation, *myself*."

It was striking that the identity doubts associated with these experiences of ghosting persisted in the present moment as interviewees recalled them:

> Frankly after the whole thing with my parents, you know, our relationship hasn't really ever recovered to be honest. It has been hard. The subtle ignoring, the no-replies, and two blue ticks [on WhatsApp] when I text my mum, and the preferential treatment my brother gets just because he is straight and I am not. It is like he can do anything he likes and just because he is straight he is still going to be a better son than me. That's how it is. It has kind of made me a bit more like dependent because I really want that love and sometimes I demand it, not just from my parents but I do it in relationships. I reckon it's because I've been feeling pretty unloved and am

> not exactly loving myself right now either. Things have got better but not completely healed, that's for sure. (Joe, gay man)

When Joe came out as gay, his parents began to distance themselves from him and he reported being ghosted by them. Ghosting did not occur in isolation—Joe noted that his parents favored his heterosexual brother with whom their behavior did not change. This interpersonal comparison made him more aware of his own isolation. The psychological effects of ghosting from his parents were manifold. On the one hand, he began to doubt his self-esteem viewing his brother as "a better son" to his parents and, on the other hand, he acknowledged the impact that this experience had on his attachment style—he reportedly became dependent upon others.

Consistent with identity process theory, individuals who experienced uncertainty and identity doubts due to their ghosting experiences attempted to cope. Despite his attempts to cope and the subsequent improvements to his wellbeing, Joe acknowledged the continued threat to self-esteem as a result of these experiences: "I've been feeling pretty unloved and am not exactly loving myself right now either." For some, the uncertainty itself impeded coping and limited the availability of effective coping strategies:

> Listen if you are told you are scum and to fuck off then, yes, fine, then the recovery can start. I've never been told that clearly. I'm just kept on a hook, like hanging, and it makes you doubt everything. You don't know if you are imagining it or if it is real. People don't understand it when you explain and I don't know how I feel about myself either. Am I a good person or not? Is my sexuality right or wrong? It has just made me confused and I wish I could force them [her grandparents] to talk it out once and for all and just to decide. (Karen, bisexual woman)

A unifying thread across participants' accounts of experiencing ghosting after coming out was the uncertainty that characterized it. Interviewees reported their inability to cope and the continued identity doubts that they experienced precisely because they did not have certainty and closure in relation to the relationship in question. Karen described her feelings of uncertainty as being "just kept on a hook, like hanging," which made her feel doubtful "about everything." She doubted her own judgment, as well as her own sense of identity: "I don't know how I feel about myself either." More specifically, her experience of ghosting in the aftermath of coming out to her family called into question her self-esteem and the value that she appended to her sexual identity, in particular. She and others referred to the uncertainty as a significant impediment to initiating the coping process following the rupture of valued relationships. For Karen, recovery could not begin until she knew the status of her relationship.

Gaslighting, Identity Doubt, and (Re)Construal

Several interviewees described some form of psychological manipulation from a significant other after they came out to them that in turn made them doubt their reality and, in some cases, their identity:

> Obviously I'm telling you how I feel like now, looking back because at the time I didn't know what people were doing to me and I just took it at face value but looking back and knowing the definition of the word "gaslighting" now I can safely say that, yes, I faced that full-on. I was told I was imagining it when I was being ignored and to just grow up. I was talked to like I was straight after clearly coming out. When I said "oh but you remember that conversation where I told you I was a lesbian" I was looked at if I was stupid. They were playing with my head and I find it pretty hard to forgive that. These are people who are meant to make me feel safe. (Jill, lesbian woman)

Upon reflection, some participants attributed the label "gaslighting" to the negative experiences that they had faced from significant others when they came out to them. Some of them had uncritically accepted manipulative behavior from significant others because it was confusing and they were uncertain about their motives. Indeed, Jill provided several examples of gaslighting when she came out to her parents, siblings, and extended family. When she confronted them about their ghosting behavior, she reportedly faced gaslighting: "I was told I was imagining it… and to grow up." It is easy to see how this might exacerbate feelings of uncertainty and confusion habitually associated with this form of psychological violence. Furthermore, Jill's sexual identity was invalidated by several significant others when she came out to them, which she perceived in terms of gaslighting: "they were playing with my head." Her coming out was conveniently "forgotten" (not acknowledged) when she mentioned it to others. In other words, she now construed her significant others' refusal to acknowledge her lesbian identity as a form of psychological manipulation—to undo what she had attempted to achieve by coming out.

Crucially, for Jill and others, these experiences of gaslighting were deemed to be distressing because they emanated from people she hoped would be accepting, understanding, and supportive:

> When people who you love start playing with your head regardless of the intentions, good or bad, it does have an effect on you and you start believing it and doubting yourself. I came out because I was ready to and because I had accepted who I was finally but then I started going back into the closet and that was the effect of what they were telling me. (Ali, gay man)

Negative experiences of coming out to people who were important were especially distressing precisely because of the expectations of acceptance, inclusion, and understanding that individuals had of their significant others. Interviewees were realistic about the challenges associated with coming out but expected their significant others to exhibit some empathy toward them when they shared such important information about their identities. As indicated in Ali's account, reported experiences of gaslighting from significant others ("people you love") could have especially negative effects. He reported doubts about his identity as he himself had begun to internalize the stigma levelled at him by people who mattered. Gaslighting caused identity doubt, on the one hand, and had a regressive effect upon his sexual identity development, on the other hand. Indeed, Ali stated that the doubts that he experienced in relation to his identity led him "back into the closet."

Similarly, other interviewees expressed the significant impact that identity doubts had on their own self-construal and coping strategies:

> The most difficult part of it is that I started to believe it or at least I wanted to believe it and then I started just playing a role and acting like I was straight but that doesn't alter the fact that I am gay so I was being a fake. (Sam, gay man)

Having derived positive meanings in relation to his gay identity, gaslighting from significant others made Sam believe the messages being relayed to him regarding his sexuality. More specifically, he reported now internalizing some of these messages, thereby undoing the identity work that he had undertaken. It was reported in Chap. 7 that some interviewees deployed the passing and role compliance strategies for coping with challenges to their identity. These interpersonal coping strategies are different from denial which is, conversely, intrapsychic in nature—Sam acknowledged "playing a role" and passing as heterosexual to avoid stigma. He and other interviewees were essentially told by their significant others that they were not really LGB and their coming out experiences were erased from the collective memory of the family. Yet, the conflict between intrapsychic self-perception and interpersonal self-presentation remained and continued to generate doubts about identity:

> My friend, at the time my best friend, started telling me that it was a normal phase and that he knew a guy who was gay and then he got a girlfriend and it was all sorted. And I respected him a lot at the time and saw him as a sort of well-wisher so it set me back a bit in my identity because I started doubting who I really was, being bi I mean, and started wondering if I was actually straight or something. Like there was a cut in how I was trying to be and my coming out was reversed because of him really. (Mike, bisexual man)

There was a recurrent theme in the interviews concerning the ways in which significant others, such as family members and close friends, attempted to construct the coming-out individual's sexuality as a transient phase or behavioral pattern to downgrade its significance. Mike's best friend attempted to substantiate his theory that "it was a normal phase" by recounting an anecdote of a male acquaintance who had come out as gay but allegedly became heterosexual and "got a girlfriend." This strategy was intended to persuade him that he was not definitely bisexual and that his sexuality could change.

In Mike's case, his best friend could exert influence upon him because Mike respected and trusted him and considered him a "well-wisher." He had high expectations of his best friend and at the time did not entertain the possibility that this could be gaslighting. Mike's account highlighted the significant psychological impact of his former best friend's behavior toward him, which he now, in retrospect, deemed to constitute gaslighting.

Like several other interviewees, Mike reported experiencing doubts about his identity and felt that his best friend's response to his coming out represented a "set back" in relation to his identity. In other words, he felt that the doubts generated by his best friend's comments in turn had a regressive effect upon his identity. Having clarified his sexual identity at the intrapsychic level, Mike subsequently began to doubt his identity in different ways. First, he expressed doubts about the content of his identity—he came out as bisexual but subsequently began to question whether he might actually be heterosexual. Second, he experienced doubt about his sense of continuity. He described discontinuity between his desired self ("how I was trying to be") and his contemporary self. Third, he described a psychological reversal of his coming out due to these comments.

In a similar vein, coming-out individuals described the power of significant others to bring about (undesirable) psychological changes in relation to their identity, which reflects gaslighting:

> I was made to think that it's all happening in my head. My mother was making out that something has gone wrong and triggered it but I'll recover, that I can't be bi because that doesn't happen in our family. It was a traumatic thing to face because the crazy thing is I started believing it for a bit. She was saying that it was all her fault but I'd recover and she'd help so of course you believe it when it's someone you really love like your own mother. I acted like from a script for a bit and it did make me feel a bit better about myself. I mean, at least I was being a better daughter to my mum and dad but you can't go on doubting yourself forever. (Deborah, bisexual woman)

A commonality across participants' accounts of gaslighting was that they were made to feel by people whom they trusted that they were imagining or misconstruing their sexuality. These trusted others indicated either explicitly or implicitly the criteria for acceptance, inclusion, and belonging. Coming-out individuals were not necessarily excluded but were essentially given a choice: either to accept the criteria or face rejection. For instance, Deborah was told "that [being bisexual] doesn't happen in our family" and was made to feel that "something has gone wrong" in relation to her sexual orientation. Her mother's claim that she could "recover" from bisexuality constructed her sexual orientation as an illness, further reinforcing the stigma appended to it. Deborah's mother was clearly stigmatizing her daughter's sexual identity but framed this as genuine concern for her wellbeing. She even took personal responsibility for her daughter's sexuality, implying that there must have been some deficiency in her parenting that had caused her daughter to become bisexual. This could be aversive for self-esteem.

Like Deborah, other interviewees reported varied strategies for coping with such threats to their identity. Some reported compliance with the expectations and prescriptions of their significant others, essentially by concealing their sexuality and by feigning heterosexuality. This could temporarily shield identity from identity hazards with the potential to undermine feelings of self-esteem. Deborah did indeed report experiencing higher self-esteem during this period and that she was "being a better daughter." However, this strategy for coping placed her in a state of identity doubt which itself is neither sustainable in the long term nor optimal for psychological wellbeing. As she noted, "you can't go doubting yourself forever."

> My grandparents brought me up and were really good parents actually and did everything for me and I truly still love them. They're from a generation that doesn't really get this and they are pretty religious so when they found out they didn't take it well and they tried to convince me that I'm not bisexual although they didn't use that word. "Bent" was the word my grandpa used. They took all the responsibility for my sexuality and me having turned out that way and it, first of all, made me think my sexuality is flawed but also it made me believe it myself which wasn't good for how I

> was feeling at the time, I won't lie. I tried to change and started just downplaying and suppressing me being bisexual because I didn't want to accept it even though I had accepted it and decided to tell the people I loved most, my grandparents. (Peter, bisexual man)

This extract too highlighted the significant impact of gaslighting upon self-perception, with those exposed to it reporting identity doubt. When Peter came out as bisexual to his grandparents, they attempted to convince him that he was mistaken about his bisexuality and that he was in fact heterosexual. Upon reflection, he remained of the view that his grandparents who acted as guardians "were really good parents" and, consequently, held them in high regard. Peter had accepted his sexual identity, but his grandparents' attempt to convince him that he was mistaken and their stigmatization of his sexuality made him doubt its value and to internalize the view that it was flawed. Like several other interviewees, he consequently concealed his bisexuality from others (which essentially reversed the identity work that he had undertaken to come out in the first place). He actively tried to change his sexual orientation to conform to the expectations of his grandparents: "the people I loved most."

Overview

This chapter describes experiences of three forms of psychological violence among coming-out LGB people: microaggressions, ghosting, and gaslighting. Overt discrimination against LGB is increasingly stigmatized but, as highlighted in previous chapters, it still occurs subtly when LGB people come out. Although there are now many studies that show the effects of microaggressions upon LGB people, there is limited empirical insight into experience of gaslighting and ghosting from significant others in the context of coming out. This chapter shows that exposure to these forms of psychological violence can induce negative changes in identity. It is associated with increased uncertainty—coming-out individuals do not know whether they are being definitively rejected, but many deduce this to be the case. The uncertainty associated with microaggressions, gaslighting, and ghosting can engender identity doubt. Due to the subtle nature of these forms of psychological violence, LGB people may find it difficult to challenge them and to seek support from others who often do not understand the psychological harm associated with these identity hazards. Moreover, in view of the identity threats associated with exposure to these hazards, coming-out individuals try to cope, often using deflective strategies, such as compliance and passing, which can have regressive effects on sexual identity development.

References

Abreu, R. L., Tyler Lefevor, G., Barrita, A. M., Gonzalez, K. A., & Watson, R. J. (2023). Intersectional microaggressions, depressive symptoms, and the role of LGBTQ-specific parental support in a sample of Latinx sexual and gender minority youth. *Journal of Adolescence, 95*(3), 584–595. https://doi.org/10.1002/jad.12139

Akdeniz, B., & Cıhan, H. (2024). Gaslighting and interpersonal relationships: Systematic review. *Psikiyatride Güncel Yaklaşımlar - Current Approaches in Psychiatry, 16*(1), 146–158.

Astleitner, H., Bains, A., & Hörmann, S. (2023). The effects of personality and social media experiences on mental health: Examining the mediating role of fear of missing out, ghosting, and vaguebooking. *Computers in Human Behavior, 138*, 107436. https://doi.org/10.1016/j.chb.2022.107436

Collins, T. J., Thomas, A.-F., & Harris, E. (2023). Unwanted and unfollowed: Defining ghosting and the role of social media unfollowing. *Personal Relationships, 30*(3), 939–959. https://doi.org/10.1111/pere.12492

Cvetkovska, S., Jaspal, R., Verkuyten, M., & Adelson, L. (2024). Coping with being tolerated: Trans experiences. *Psychology of Sexual Orientation and Gender Diversity, 11*(1), 31–41. https://doi.org/10.1037/sgd0000580

DeSon, J. J., & Andover, M. S. (2024). Microaggressions toward sexual and gender minority emerging adults: An updated systematic review of psychological correlates and outcomes and the role of intersectionality. *LGBT Health, 11*(4), 249–268. https://doi.org/10.1089/lgbt.2023.0032

Dorri, A. A., Stone, A. L., Heffington, B. I., Njowo, P. J., Rivera, G., Schnarrs, P. W., & Salcido, R. (2024). "We're not gonna talk about this, it didn't happen. You're confused": Adverse communication in family responses to mental health, childhood sexual assault, and LGBTQ identities. *Society and Mental Health, 14*(1), 39–55. https://doi.org/10.1177/21568693231170901

Forrai, M., Koban, K., & Matthews, J. (2023). Short-sighted ghosts. Psychological antecedents and consequences of ghosting others within emerging adults' romantic relationships and friendships. *Telematics and Informatics, 80*, 101969. https://doi.org/10.1016/j.tele.2023.101969

Freedman, G., Hales, A. H., Powell, D. N., Le, B., & Williams, K. D. (2022). The role of gender and safety concerns in romantic rejection decisions. *Journal of Experimental Social Psychology, 102*, 1–12. https://doi.org/10.1016/j.jesp.2022.104368

Freedman, G., Powell, D. N., Le, B., & Williams, K. D. (2024). Emotional experiences of ghosting. *Journal of Social Psychology, 164*(3), 367–386. https://doi.org/10.1080/00224545.2022.2081528

Güleç, S., & Özbay, A. (2024). Psychological resilience, gaslighting and life satisfaction in a sample of Turkish women. *Women's Studies International Forum, 105*, 102945. https://doi.org/10.1016/j.wsif.2024.102945

Hailes, H. P., & Goodman, L. A. (2025). "They're out to take away your sanity": A qualitative investigation of gaslighting in intimate partner violence. *Journal of Family Violence, 40*(2), 269–282. https://psycnet.apa.org/doi/10.1007/s10896-023-00652-1

Jaspal, R. (2017). Coping with ethnic prejudice on the gay scene: British South Asian gay men. *Journal of LGBT Youth, 14*(2), 172–190. https://doi.org/10.1080/19361653.2016.1264907

Jaspal, R., & Lopes, B. (2025a). Vulnerability to "breadcrumbing" in a sample of adults in the United Kingdom: A cross-sectional survey study. *Psychology International, 7*(3), 71. https://doi.org/10.3390/psycholint7030071

Jaspal, R., & Lopes, B. (2025b). Exposure to ghosting, gaslighting and coercion in religious and non-religious people in the United Kingdom. *Mental Health, Religion and Culture*. https://doi.org/10.1080/13674676.2025.2524402

Jaspal, R., & Nerlich, B. (2017). Polarised reporting about HIV prevention: Social representations of pre-exposure prophylaxis (PrEP) in the UK press. *Health: An Interdisciplinary Journal for the Social Study of Health, Illness and Medicine, 21*(5), 478–497. https://doi.org/10.1177/1363459316649763

Johnson, V. E., Nadal, K. L., Sissoko, D. R. G., & King, R. (2021). "It's not in your head": Gaslighting, 'splaining, victim blaming, and other harmful reactions to microaggressions. *Perspectives on Psychological Science, 16*(5), 1024–1036. https://doi.org/10.1177/17456916211011963

Jolley, D., & Jaspal, R. (2020). Discrimination, HIV conspiracy theories and pre-exposure prophylaxis acceptability in gay men. *Sexual Health, 17*(6), 525–533. https://doi.org/10.1071/SH20154

Kaufman, T. M. L., Baams, L., & Dubas, J. S. (2017). Microaggressions and depressive symptoms in sexual minority youth: The roles of rumination and social support. *Psychology of Sexual Orientation and Gender Diversity, 4*(2), 184–192. https://doi.org/10.1037/sgd0000219

Kim, S., Warren, E., Jahangir, T., Al-Garadi, M., Guo, Y., Yang, Y. C., Lakamana, S., & Sarker, A. (2023). Characteristics of intimate partner violence and survivor's needs during the COVID-19 pandemic: Insights from subreddits related to intimate partner violence. *Journal of Interpersonal Violence, 38*(17–18), 9693–9716. https://doi.org/10.1177/08862605231168816

Konings, F., Sumter, S., & Vandenbosch, L. (2023). It's not you, it's me: Experiences with ghosting on mobile dating applications and Belgian emerging adults' self-esteem. *Sexuality and Culture, 27*(11), 1328–1351. https://doi.org/10.1007/s12119-023-10065-3

Leckfor, C. M., Wood, N. R., Slatcher, R. B., & Hales, A. H. (2023). From close to ghost: Examining the relationship between the need for closure, intentions to ghost, and reactions to being Ghosted. *Journal of Social and Personal Relationships, 40*(8), 2422–2444. https://doi.org/10.1177/02654075221149955

LeFebvre, L. E., Rasner, R. D., & Allen, M. (2019). "I guess I'll never know...": Noninitiators account-making after being ghosted. *Journal of Loss and Trauma, 25*(5), 395–415. https://doi.org/10.1080/15325024.2019.1694299

Legge, M. M., Flanders, C. E., & Robinson, M. (2018). Young bisexual people's experiences of microaggression: Implications for social work. *Social Work in Mental Health, 16*(2), 125–144. https://doi.org/10.1080/15332985.2017.1357669

Li, Y., & Samp, J. A. (2023). Gaslighting LGBTQ+ individuals: Correlates of gaslighting experiences, gaslighters' characteristics, and gaslighting techniques. *Communication Studies, 74*(4), 356–376. https://doi.org/10.1080/10510974.2023.2209605

Lomash, E. F., Brown, T. D., & Paz Galupo, M. (2019). "A whole bunch of love the sinner hate the sin": LGBTQ microaggressions experienced in religious and spiritual context. *Journal of Homosexuality, 66*(10), 1495–1511. https://doi.org/10.1080/00918369.2018.1542204

Lopes, B., & Jaspal, R. (2025). Exposure to ghosting, gaslighting and coercion and mental health outcomes. *Partner Abuse.* https://doi.org/10.1891/PA-2024-0031

Marchi, M., Travascio, A., Uberti, D., De Micheli, E., Quartaroli, F., Laquatra, G., et al. (2024). Microaggression toward LGBTIQ people and implications for mental health: A systematic review. *The International Journal of Social Psychiatry, 70*(1), 23–35. https://doi.org/10.1177/00207640231194478

Matsick, J. L., & Rubin, J. D. (2018). Bisexual prejudice among lesbian and gay people: Examining the roles of gender and perceived sexual orientation. *Psychology of Sexual Orientation and Gender Diversity, 5*(2), 143–155. https://doi.org/10.1037/sgd0000283

McCabe, P. C., Dragowski, E. A., & Rubinson, F. (2013). What is homophobic bias anyway? Defining and recognizing microaggressions and harassment of LGBTQ youth. *Journal of School Violence, 12*(1), 7–26. https://doi.org/10.1080/15388220.2012.731664

McInroy, L. B., Beer, O. W. J., Scheadler, T. R., Craig, S. L., & Eaton, A. D. (2024). Exploring the psychological and physiological impacts of digital microaggressions and hostile online climates on LGBTQ + youth. *Current Psychology, 43*(3), 2586–2596. https://doi.org/10.1007/s12144-023-04435-1

Mendoza-Pérez, J. C., Trejo-Hernández, J. C., Olmedo-Neri, R. A., Vega-Cauich, J. I., Lozano-Verduzco, I., & Craig, S. (2024). Microaggressions based on sexual orientation and the mental health of gay men youth in three Mexican Cities. *Journal of LGBT Youth, 21*(3), 469–489. https://doi.org/10.1080/19361653.2023.2185336

Nadal, K. L. Y. (2023). *Dismantling everyday discrimination: Microaggressions toward LGBTQ people*. American Psychological Association. https://doi.org/10.1037/0000335-001

Nadal, K. L., Wong, Y., Issa, M. A., Meterko, V., Leon, J., & Wideman, M. (2011). Sexual orientation microaggressions: Processes and coping mechanisms for lesbian, gay, and bisexual individuals. *Journal of LGBT Issues in Counseling, 5*(1), 21–46. https://doi.org/10.1080/15538605.2011.554606

Navarro, R., Larrañaga, E., Yubero, S., & Víllora, B. (2020). Psychological correlates of ghosting and breadcrumbing experiences: A preliminary study among adults. *International Journal of Environmental Research and Public Health, 17*(3), 1116. https://doi.org/10.3390/ijerph17031116

Pancani, L., Aureli, N., & Riva, P. (2022). Relationship dissolution strategies: Comparing the psychological consequences of ghosting, orbiting, and rejection. *Cyberpsychology: Journal of Psychosocial Research on Cyberspace, 16*(2), 9. https://doi.org/10.5817/CP2022-2-9

Pancani, L., Mazzoni, D., Aureli, N., & Riva, P. (2021). Ghosting and orbiting: An analysis of victims' experiences. *Journal of Social and Personal Relationships, 38*(7), 1987–2007. https://doi.org/10.1177/02654075211000417

Resnick, C. A., & Galupo, M. P. (2019). Assessing experiences with LGBT microaggressions in the workplace: Development and validation of the Microaggression Experiences at Work Scale. *Journal of Homosexuality, 66*(10), 1380–1403. https://doi.org/10.1080/00918369.2018.1542207

Robinson, J. L., & Rubin, L. J. (2016). Homonegative microaggressions and posttraumatic stress symptoms. *Journal of Gay & Lesbian Mental Health, 20*(1), 57–69. https://doi.org/10.1080/19359705.2015.1066729

Sadika, B., Wiebe, E., Morrison, M. A., & Morrison, T. G. (2020). Intersectional microaggressions and social support for LGBTQ persons of color: A systematic review of the Canadian-based empirical literature. *Journal of GLBT Family Studies, 16*(2), 111–147. https://doi.org/10.1080/1550428X.2020.1724125

Silva, W. A. D., Do Bú, E. A., Brito, T. R. d. S., de Figueiredo, C. V., & Pereira, C. R. (2025). The impact of sexual orientation microaggressions on the mental health of Brazilian lesbian, gay, and bisexual individuals. *Psychology of Sexual Orientation and Gender Diversity.* https://doi.org/10.1037/sgd0000807

Smith, A. U., Bostwick, W. B., Burke, L., Hequembourg, A. L., Santuzzi, A., & Hughes, T. L. (2023). How deep is the cut? The influence of daily microaggressions on bisexual women's health. *Psychology of Sexual Orientation and Gender Diversity, 10*(4), 535–548. https://doi.org/10.1037/sgd0000556

Sorrell, S. A., Lefevor, G. T., Bell, J. H., Berg, C. O., & Skidmore, S. J. (2024a). "You're not gay; You're a child of god": Microaggressions experienced by LGBTQ+ teens and their parents in the Church of Jesus Christ of Latter-Day Saints. *Family Process, 63*(1), 243–264. https://doi.org/10.1111/famp.12863

Sorrell, S. A., Lefevor, G. T., & Berg, C. O. (2024b). "Like little knives, stabbing me": The impact of microaggressions on LGBTQ+ teens and their parents in the Church of Jesus Christ of Latter-Day Saints. *Journal for the Scientific Study of Religion, 63*(2), 213–239. https://doi.org/10.1111/jssr.12882

Sterzing, P. R., & Gartner, R. E. (2020). LGBTQ Microaggressions and microaffirmations in families: Scale development and validation study. *Journal of Homosexuality, 67*(5), 600–619. https://doi.org/10.1080/00918369.2018.1553350

Swann, G., Minshew, R., Newcomb, M. E., & Mustanski, B. (2016). Validation of the Sexual Orientation Microaggression Inventory in two diverse samples of LGBTQ youth. *Archives of Sexual Behavior, 45*(6), 1289–1298. https://doi.org/10.1007/s10508-016-0718-2

Tran, D., Sullivan, C. T., & Nicholas, L. (2023). Lateral violence and microaggressions in the LGBTQ+ community: A scoping review. *Journal of Homosexuality, 70*(7), 1310–1324. https://doi.org/10.1080/00918369.2021.2020543

Wike, T., Tomlinson, C. A., Wagaman, A., Matijczak, A., Murphy, J., Watts, K., et al. (2023). The role of thwarted belongingness on the relationship between microaggressions and mental health for LGBTQ+ emerging adults. *Journal of Youth Studies, 26*(2), 286–303. https://doi.org/10.1080/13676261.2021.2010687

Winberg, C., Coleman, T., Woodford, M. R., McKie, R. M., Travers, R., & Renn, K. A. (2019). Hearing "that's so gay" and "no homo" on campus and substance use among sexual minority college students. *Journal of Homosexuality, 66*(10), 1472–1494. https://doi.org/10.1080/00918369.2018.1542208

Woodford, M. R., Chonody, J. M., Kulick, A., Brennan, D. J., & Renn, K. (2015). The LGBQ Microaggressions on Campus Scale: A scale development and validation study. *Journal of Homosexuality, 62*(12), 1660–1687. https://doi.org/10.1080/00918369.2015.1078205

Wozolek, B. (2018). Gaslighting queerness: Schooling as a place of violent assemblages. *Journal of LGBT Youth, 15*(4), 319–338. https://doi.org/10.1080/19361653.2018.1484839

Wright, A. J., & Wegner, R. T. (2012). Homonegative microaggressions and their impact on LGB individuals: A measure validity study. *Journal of LGBT Issues in Counseling, 6*(1), 34–54. https://doi.org/10.1080/15538605.2012.648578

Wu, K., & Bamishigbin, O. (2023). When silence speaks louder than words: Exploring the experiences and attitudes of ghosters. *Personal Relationships, 30*(4), 1358–1382. https://doi.org/10.1111/pere.12518

10

Coming Out in the Future

The purpose of this book was to examine the psychological aspects of coming out with a particular focus on its implications for identity processes. Written and interview accounts from over 500 lesbian, gay, and bisexual (LGB) people with diverse backgrounds showed significant variation in their experiences. Yet, there were some key commonalities across their accounts. First, it is clear that coming out matters to LGB people, especially when it involves somebody significant. Coming out is important because sexual identity itself is important (cf. Savin-Williams, 2005). LGB people may not foreground their sexual identity in all contexts but it clearly constitutes a meaningful element of identity. The accounts from LGB people shared in this book provide a powerful rebuttal to the post-gay argument that coming out no longer matters. Second, coming out can have important effects for identity processes, and identity processes in turn appear to shape the individual's decision-making about coming out. Third, there are shared social and psychological factors that appear to enhance or disrupt the coming out process, regardless of whether one self-identifies as lesbian, gay, or bisexual. These factors are articulated in the integrative theoretical framework outlined in this chapter.

R. Jaspal, *The Psychology of Coming Out*,
https://doi.org/10.1007/978-3-032-02599-9_10

Examining the Antecedents, Consequences, and Experiences of Coming Out

Based upon existing theory and research and, particularly, the findings from the two empirical studies presented in this book, an integrative theoretical framework for examining the antecedents, consequences, and experiences of coming out as LGB is proposed. The integrative theoretical framework, which builds upon the model predicting degree of outness outlined in Chap. 2, emphasizes the dynamic, reciprocal inter-relations between stimuli (identity hazards and social support), identity processes, and coming out. There are two key differences between the sexual identity development models reviewed in Chap. 2 and the integrative theoretical framework presented here that should be emphasized.

- The integrative theoretical framework attempts to explain the inter-relations between the interpersonal process of coming out and intra-psychic identity processes (focusing not only on sexual identity but on the total identity of the individual).
- It views coming out as a life-long process that occurs repeatedly across both time and space, in novel contexts, and to varying degrees with cumulative effects for the total identity of the individual and, consequently, for future coming out decision-making.

The major tenets of the theoretical framework are outlined in Fig. 10.1.

LGB people come out in particular social contexts. Some social contexts are more affirmative of their sexuality than others. Yet, the coming-out individual is tacitly aware that they are revealing an element of their identity that remains stigmatized in heteronormative societies. Part of this stigma is associated with the fact that LGB people constitute a minority—their sexuality is a marker of their difference from others (Frost & Meyer, 2023). LGB people differ in their level of exposure to identity hazards. Identity hazards have the capacity to cause damage to identity, but individuals differ in the extent to which they actually experience an identity hazard as threatening for identity. As shown in the accounts of

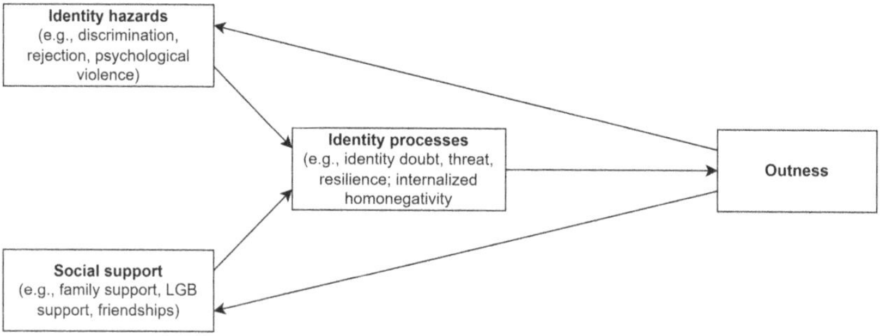

Fig. 10.1 An integrative theoretical framework for examining the antecedents, consequences, and experiences of coming out

LGB people, identity hazards include exposure to negative social representations of one's sexuality, and experiences of discrimination, rejection, invalidation, emotional distance, ambiguous loss, silencing, microaggressions, gaslighting, and ghosting due to one's sexual identity. Some of these identity hazards are overtly discriminatory and would be recognized as such by most people. Others are subtler, more difficult to detect, but no less insidious in their effects. In societies in which overt discrimination due to sexual identity is stigmatized, such as the United Kingdom, subtler identity hazards (e.g., microaggressions, emotional distance) appear to be particularly significant.

Social support refers to the perception that support from others exists and that it is available to the individual. It reflects not only the individual's perception that they are currently supported but also that they will continue to be supported in the future. It is important to note that the objective availability of social support is not the focus here. After all, an individual may be surrounded by supportive others but not perceive this support to be available to them, and some may refrain from capitalizing on support despite its availability (Jaspal & Lopes, 2025a). Rather, the focus in this book is on the *subjective perception* of support from others (Jaspal & Breakwell, 2025). The LGB people whose accounts are presented in this book described many forms of perceived social support, including family support, support from other LGB people, friendships, and romantic relationships.

Exposure to identity hazards and the perception of social support can activate various changes in identity. These changes concern not only the content of identity but also the processes underpinning identity. The term "identity processes" is used because all these changes relate, in one way or another, to the identity processes of assimilation-accommodation and evaluation (see Chap. 3). In this book, it has been shown that exposure to identity hazards and the derivation of social support are associated with many different changes to identity processes.

Exposure to identity hazards was found to be associated with the onset of internalized homonegativity (essentially the negative evaluation of sexual identity), doubts about the content of identity ("am I really LGB?"), as well as doubts about the principles that habitually guide identity processes (i.e., self-esteem, self-efficacy, continuity, and positive distinctiveness). In some cases, identity hazards appeared to generate actual threats to identity, which is harmful for psychological wellbeing. Conversely, feeling supported by others and, especially, by significant others was generally associated with a more favorable conception of one's sexual identity—this can bolster feelings of self-esteem, self-efficacy, continuity, and positive distinctiveness. As such, positive reactions to coming out that foreground one's access to support may enhance the LGB person's identity resilience over time. Indeed, there is evidence from previous research that social support predicts identity resilience (e.g., Jaspal & Breakwell, 2025).

The integrative theoretical framework proposes that it is the changes that occur in identity (and specifically to the assimilation-accommodation and evaluation processes) that in turn determine LGB people's cognition, affect, and behavior in relation to coming out. The case studies presented in Chap. 1 and the accounts presented in Chaps. 5–9 exhibit the sheer diversity of coming out experiences at both the intragroup level (among lesbian women, gay men, bisexual men, and bisexual women) and the intrapersonal level (in each individual's repertoire of coming out experiences).

Any given individual may have a positive coming out experience, followed by a negative one. Even the same coming out experience may have both positive and negative features. Some positive features of the coming out experience may generate unforeseen negative sequelae. Similarly, negative features may facilitate growth in the individual and their significant others. A positive feature may supersede a negative one, and a negative feature may overshadow a positive one. Exposure to a hazard and the derivation of social support from a significant other (i.e., a person that matters to the coming-out individual) appears to have the greatest capacity to engender changes in identity processes. Significant others constitute a wide range of people—for most participants in the studies, these significant others happened to be their parents but some also referred to other people that mattered to them.

The coming-out individual habitually experiences a combination of both hazards and social support across their coming out experiences. Some experiences may be characterized by more hazards than support; others by more support than hazards. There is thus an overall combined effect of hazards and perceived social support upon identity processes. For instance, some LGB people are clearly supported by their significant others when they come out but may also be exposed to identity hazards, such as the silencing of their LGB identity in the extended family. Perceived social support in that coming out situation may militate against the identity hazard, reducing its overall effect upon identity processes. As such, social support can be viewed as a protective factor.

The sexual identity development models generally postulate that LGB people pass through a linear set of developmental processes, incrementally constructing a positive sexual identity. The lack of clarity about movement between the stages has been noted as a limitation. Based on LGB people's accounts, the integrative theoretical framework posits that coming out is a dynamic process. Some specific observations can be made:

- A cumulation of identity hazards with limited or no social support can lead to identity regression (see Kroger et al., 2010 for a discussion of identity status change) to early stages of sexual identity development. For instance, a LGB person who has derived identity pride may internalize homonegativity, relive the threats to psychological coherence in relation to their sexuality and other identity elements (e.g., religion), or return to the closet when exposed to identity hazards from a significant other.

- A cumulation of supportive responses from significant others can, conversely, boost the individual's identity resilience, militate against internalized homonegativity, clarify identity doubts, and alleviate identity threat. The negative effects of future exposure to identity hazards may be greatly reduced, thereby enabling the individual to come out to others.
- The integrative theoretical framework refers to a feedback loop, with each subsequent coming out experience potentially exposing the individual to novel identity hazards or perceived social support. These novel stimuli will be perceived partly through the lens of previous experiences. Exposure to hazards and/or support precipitate further identity changes which in turn will determine future coming-out decision-making as the individual encounters novel contexts and situations.

As shown in the case studies and accounts presented in this book, LGB people who have come out to somebody significant and received support, even in the presence of identity hazards, may develop a more positive self-conception, feelings of competence and control and, thus, the capacity to come out to others. Conversely, those who encounter negative reactions with limited support may themselves internalize the stigma to which they are exposed, question their continued membership of other relevant groups, and, in some cases, return to the closet. Yet, a recurrent theme throughout this book is that LGB people tend to be resourceful and strategic in managing their coming out, choosing to do so in ways and to people that are likely to enhance, rather than threaten, the principled operation of identity processes.

Identity Pressures

When asked to reflect upon a coming out experience to a significant other, individuals described a plethora of inter-connected events and experiences, divergent emotions, and competing thoughts. Any given coming out experience may itself consist of a multitude of stimuli (i.e., identity hazards and social support). In their quest to optimize identity processes, the coming-out individual exposed to multiple stimuli appears to derive some respite from the support they receive. This was evident in some coming-out individuals' recognition and acceptance that initial reactions to their coming out might not be wholly positive. The hope that they would be supported provided some psychological relief. However, it should be acknowledged that confirmation bias is also likely to play a role in meaning-making (Hart et al., 2009). For instance, a LGB person with existing internalized homonegativity and thus a negative belief about their own sexuality may be prone to focus on the identity hazards (confirming their own prior beliefs) from significant others (Breakwell & Jaspal, 2022). Conversely, a person with high identity resilience may be primed to believe that they still have personal and social worth, are competent and in control, and so on, despite exposure to identity hazards (Breakwell, 2021).

Identity process theory posits that human beings strive for feelings of self-esteem, self-efficacy, continuity, and positive distinctiveness—these principles are said to guide the identity processes of assimilation-accommodation and evaluation (Jaspal & Breakwell, 2014). The accounts presented in this book show that, in the context of coming out at least, the motives for authenticity, belonging, and psychological coherence are also significant. These can be considered identity principles in their own right, since they appear to add greater explanatory power to identity construction, management, and protection in coming-out LGB people (see Breakwell, 2014). Incidentally, authenticity, belonging, and psychological coherence have been discussed in previous research. Markowe (1996, 2002) outlined the significance of authenticity and affiliation/belonging in lesbian women's sexual identity development, and Jaspal and Cinnirella (2010, 2012, 2014) have shown the role of psychological coherence in the management of sexuality and religion among gay men of religious faith. They appear also to be central to LGB people's decision-making about coming out.

Individuals emphasized the role of coming out in facilitating feelings of authenticity. In many cases, this appeared to be a key motive for coming out and coming out was deemed to be a success when it produced feelings of authenticity. Conversely, one of the main fears cited by coming-out individuals was the loss of acceptance, inclusion, and support from significant others and, especially, their immediate family members. In some cases, these fears were realized. As such, belonging appeared to operate as a motive for concealing their sexual identity from significant others. When threatened, belonging was sometimes sought from other sources, such as an alternative "chosen family." Some individuals also reported returning to the closet, essentially reversing their coming out, in order to salvage feelings of belonging.

This book repeatedly refers to the total identity of the coming-out individual. After all, the identity of the coming-out individual consists not only of their sexuality but of many other elements. Some of these elements may be deemed to be irrelevant to sexuality. Others become relevant and are thus said to be "inter-connected" with sexuality (Jaspal & Cinnirella, 2010). Identity process theory refers not only to the assimilation of novel elements but also their accommodation in the identity structure. It is therefore essential to understand how other elements deemed to be inter-connected with one's sexuality might impinge upon coming out.

All too often the role of other identity elements is overlooked and the coming-out individual is viewed exclusively in terms of their sexual identity. This approach limits our understanding of the psychological aspects of coming out. Some participants in the studies reported here were of religious faith and believed that coming out as LGB would, and in some cases did, imperil their religious identity. Many others construed their sexuality to be at odds with their family identity. These other identity elements were thus key considerations in some people's coming-out decision-making. They shaped how coming out was performed and the extent to which they came out and remained out. Essentially, the coming-out individual is motivated to develop or retain feelings of compatibility and coherence between identity elements that, for whatever reason, become inter-connected.

It is thus important to note the significance of authenticity, belonging, and psychological coherence, in addition to the other identity principles, in relation to coming out. The relationship between the principles that guide the operation of identity processes requires some clarification. The data suggest that coming out may be challenging due partly to competing identity pressures. The enhancement of one identity principle may produce doubts about another. For instance, the quest for continuity between one's self-conception and self-presentation as gay may inadvertently produce threats to self-esteem due to the social stigma associated with gay identity. The desire for authenticity as a lesbian may, in some contexts, be at odds with the motive to belong, since coming out and living authentically as a lesbian may lead to exclusion from the family. Some LGB people cope with these competing identity pressures by focusing on their intrapsychic authenticity (i.e., feeling authentic) rather than their interpersonal authenticity (i.e., through self-presentation). Incidentally, the reality of identity pressures is acknowledged in optimal distinctiveness theory (Brewer, 1991), which posits that individuals seek to strike an optimal balance between the competing motives to be distinctive and to belong in social groups. The pressures between the identity principles in relation to coming out must be a key consideration in supporting LGB people.

Furthermore, the coping strategies deployed by coming-out individuals to limit the negative effects of identity hazards, either pre-emptively or reactively, may create threats of their own. This represents another identity pressure associated with coming out. For instance, passing as heterosexual may alleviate threats to self-esteem but undermine feelings of authenticity. Negativism toward those who generate identity hazards may protect continuity but curtail feelings of belonging. Sexual identity concealment may safeguard belonging but damage continuity. Coming-out individuals are resourceful in using the strategies that are available to them in any given context. Yet, coping has its limits (Breakwell, 1986; Jaspal & Lopes, 2025b). In some cases, the identity pressures may appear to be irreconcilable, leading to identity threat and, as seen in participants' accounts, to significant psychological distress. The key is to increase the availability of social support in its many guises, as well as other adaptive, effective, and sustainable coping strategies that can enhance identity processes.

The accounts presented in this book should be considered with one caveat in mind. A limitation associated with the elicitation of data that relies upon recall of a past event is that recall occurs retrospectively through the lens of the individual's present identity. In other words, the individual may recall that experience in ways that do not disrupt the principled operation of identity processes. As they recall their past experiences, they are subject to identity pressures in the present. They may attempt to make sense of a past event so that it fits within their overall life narrative, in order to safeguard feelings of continuity (Addis & Tippett, 2008). Social desirability biases may be activated to protect self-esteem (Robins et al., 2001). Past coping strategies reliant upon deflection may have completely erased threatening events from memory. Current pressures to maintain self-esteem, self-efficacy, continuity, and positive distinctiveness may influence one's recollection of the past. Notwithstanding these limitations, coming-out individuals' accounts powerfully demonstrate the lasting effects of coming out experiences for identity processes, with the potential to shape current and future decision-making (see also Ryan et al., 2015).

Supporting Coming-Out Lesbian, Gay, and Bisexual People

LGB people approach the prospect of coming out with varying levels of perceived readiness to do so. They vary in their levels of identity resilience, perceived social support, and exposure to identity hazards. This diversity is shown throughout this book. Therefore, it is problematic to assume that all LGB people should come out in a traditional sense, or that they should come out in the same way and to the same extent. The variation in coming out reflects the diversity of the identities of LGB people themselves. The LGB people whose accounts are reproduced in this book were based in the United Kingdom but some of the identity hazards faced by those in other cultures and societies were discussed in Chap. 1. This diversity must be acknowledged. The dominant social representation of coming out that constructs it as the only means of being authentic must be reframed. Crucially, the stigmatization of LGB people who are in the closet should be challenged. In essence, LGB people should not feel pressured to come out due to these social pressures or in ways that are incompatible with their identity.

Some specific recommendations can be offered for supporting LGB people to come out if they choose to do so:

- The dominant social representation that links authenticity to outness has been discussed. The LGB person should be introduced to a broad range of social representations of coming out that acknowledge the varying degrees of outness and the various ways in which authenticity and indeed other identity principles can be derived. Moreover, exposure to alternative ways of viewing coming out may provide greater flexibility in relation to coming out and LGB people may thus be better positioned to come out strategically (Orne, 2011), that is, in ways that enhance identity processes.
- The derivation of social support is key. LGB people must be able to access social support in order to reduce the risks associated with exposure to identity hazards. This is important because these hazards not only continue to exist but are manifested in increasingly subtle ways (e.g., microaggressions, ghosting, gaslighting, and invalidation). The derivation of social support depends upon at least some self-disclosure. Social support comes in many different forms. The most appropriate source of social support for each individual will depend on that individual's own identity (Jaspal & Lopes, 2025b). For some, this may be involvement in the LGB community and, for others, this may be engagement with a sibling, a therapist, or religious group. In societies that are not affirmative of LGB identities, social contact on the Internet may be deemed to be preferable. Bearing in mind the entirety of their identity (consisting of multiple elements), the LGB person should be supported to identify and access the most appropriate support for them.
- Identity resilience is an important determinant of adaptive coping and of psychological wellbeing. People can be supported to build feelings of identity resilience through psychotherapeutic intervention (Breakwell, 2021; Jaspal, 2018). Morrow (2004) provides some guidelines for interventions with LGB people who are contemplating coming out. She recommends that the clients' stage of sexual identity development be assessed and that their knowledge base regarding sexual issues be developed. She notes the importance of preparing the

client for potential upheaval following their coming out. Supporting the client to enhance their identity resilience would also be valuable.
- In this book, a distinction is made between the experience of identity doubt and that of identity threat (Chap. 3). This distinction was observable in the accounts of the LGB people shared in this book. Both identity doubt and identity threat appear to be impediments to coming out. Social support and other adaptive coping strategies are likely to be most effective when the individual is experiencing identity doubt rather than full-blown threat. It is at that stage that intervention would be most useful since doubts can be resolved more easily than actual threat through, for instance, the derivation of social support.

The focus of this book is on the interpersonal process of coming out to significant others. The identity hazards and support with the greatest capacity to influence identity processes come from the coming-out individual's significant others. Their social representations of LGB people and reactions to coming out must be a focus for future interventions designed to support LGB people before, during, and after coming out. In view of the significant threats to identity that can be produced by identity hazards, it may be tempting to denigrate the originators of these hazards. This would be unproductive. Rather, it is important to identify ways in which the significant others of coming-out individuals can be supported to be supportive.

Most respondents in the studies focused on their experiences of coming out to their families. The following recommendations therefore focus on families but may be transferable to other groups significant to the coming-out individual:

- Therapeutic interventions for supporting families with coming out should acknowledge the risk of identity threat in significant others. Jaspal (2020) conducted an interview study of 12 British South Asian people whose sons had come out as gay. The "conversational enquiries" conducted revealed three main themes. Parents appeared to experience threats to their sense of self-esteem and continuity upon learning that their son was gay. They acknowledged that denial (of their son's gay identity or of the significance of their identity) had been their preferred coping strategy in response to their coming out. Parents used self-isolation in conjunction with denial in order to avoid social stigma from others in their cultural environment. Existing empowerment models (e.g., Matthews & Salazar, 2012) outline strategies and interventions for families, such as enhancing awareness of LGB issues, acknowledging personal prejudices, addressing family, cultural, religious, and other social issues, and providing access to resources that can provide clients with support with coming out. Significant others must be supported to elect adaptive strategies for coping with their own threat, which in turn may enable them to be more supportive toward coming-out individuals.

- In an article focusing on the support organization PFLAG (Parents, Friends, and Family of Lesbians and Gays), Broad (2011) notes that the organization acknowledges the grief experienced by many parents but offers the promise of displacing these negative feelings through a focus on love for the coming-out individual. This can be achieved partly by facilitating access to social support among the significant others of coming-out individuals through such organizations (Saltzburg, 2009). When significant others have resolved threats to their own identity, a refocus on the coming-out individual's identity may enable them to become more effective supporters.
- Social support and the resolution of threats to identity, both in the coming-out individual and their significant others, are contingent upon effective communication (Allen, 2022). The accounts presented in this book highlight the significance of silence as an impediment to coping. Negative parental reactions to coming out can be attributed to the absence of family resources to deal with the coming-out situation, most notably effective communication skills (Baiocco et al., 2015). LaSala (2000) highlights the value of developing noncombative communication skills during the coming out event. Interventions to enhance communication skills would enable both coming-out individuals and their significant others to address each other's emotional needs, derive support from one another, and, potentially, to develop the positive interpersonal relations described in Chap. 6.

Conclusion

The accounts, case studies, and previous theory and research presented in this book collectively provide a compelling argument against the notion that LGB people now live in a post-gay era in which coming out no longer matters. Sexual identities matter and so does coming out. Many of the identity hazards faced by LGB people may be more subtle in their presentation but are no less insidious in their psychological effects. Social support appears to militate against identity hazards, facilitating the construction, management, and protection of identity when coming out. Coming out should not be viewed as a singular event. It is in fact a lifelong process that never ceases. Coming out happens in many different ways and to varying degrees. Identity processes shape the coming out process, and coming out in turn shapes identity processes. In addition to the recommendations for supporting coming-out LGB people and their significant others, there is a societal challenge that we can collectively address: the eradication of anti-LGB stigma in all its guises and manifestations. LGB people of course come out in social contexts. We collectively create those social contexts. We thus have the power to make them affirmative of the total identity of the coming-out individual.

References

Addis, D. R., & Tippett, L. J. (2008). The contributions of autobiographical memory to the content and continuity of identity: A social-cognitive neuroscience approach. In F. Sani (Ed.), *Self-continuity: Individual and collective perspectives* (pp. 71–84). Psychology Press.

Allen, J. L. (2022). "And then I came out…": A thematic analysis of gay men's recalled memories of coming out and its impact on their mental health and well-being. *Journal of Gay & Lesbian Social Services, 35*(4), 488–510. https://doi.org/10.1080/10538720.2022.2140242

Baiocco, R., Fontanesi, L., Santamaria, F., Ioverno, S., Marasco, B., Baumgartner, E., Willoughby, B. L. B., & Laghi, F. (2015). Negative parental responses to coming out and family functioning in a sample of lesbian and gay young adults. *Journal of Child and Family Studies, 24*(5), 1490–1500. https://doi.org/10.1007/s10826-014-9954-z

Breakwell, G. M. (1986). *Coping with threatened identities*. Methuen.

Breakwell, G. M. (2014). Identity and social representations. In R. Jaspal & G. M. Breakwell (Eds.), *Identity process theory* (pp. 118–134). Cambridge University Press.

Breakwell, G. M. (2021). Identity resilience: Its origins in identity processes and its role in coping with threat. *Contemporary Social Science, 16*(5), 573–588. https://doi.org/10.1080/21582041.2021.1999488

Breakwell, G. M., & Jaspal, R. (2022). Coming out, distress, and identity threat in gay men in the United Kingdom. *Sexuality Research & Social Policy, 19*(3), 1166–1177. https://doi.org/10.1007/s13178-021-00608-4

Brewer, M. B. (1991). The social self: On being the same and different at the same time. *Personality and Social Psychology Bulletin, 17*(5), 475–482. https://doi.org/10.1177/0146167291175001

Broad, K. L. (2011). Coming out for parents, families and friends of lesbians and gays: From support group grieving to love advocacy. *Sexualities, 14*(4), 399–415. https://doi.org/10.1177/1363460711406792

Frost, D. M., & Meyer, I. H. (2023). Minority stress theory: Application, critique, and continued relevance. *Current Opinion in Psychology, 51*, 101579. https://doi.org/10.1016/j.copsyc.2023.101579

Hart, W., Albarracín, D., Eagly, A. H., Brechan, I., Lindberg, M. J., & Merrill, L. (2009). Feeling validated versus being correct: A meta-analysis of selective exposure to information. *Psychological Bulletin, 135*(4), 555–588. https://doi.org/10.1037/a0015701

Jaspal, R. (2018). *Enhancing sexual health, self-identity and wellbeing among men who have sex with men: A guide for practitioners*. Jessica Kingsley Publishers.

Jaspal, R. (2020). Parental reactions to British South Asian young men who identify as gay. *Journal of GLBT Family Studies, 16*(4), 402–417. https://doi.org/10.1080/1550428X.2019.1684412

Jaspal, R., & Breakwell, G. M. (2025). Fear during crises: The roles of perceived risk, appraisal support and identity resilience. *Journal of Risk Research, 28*(1), 17–31. https://doi.org/10.1080/13669877.2025.2485048

Jaspal, R., & Cinnirella, M. (2010). Coping with potentially incompatible identities: Accounts of religious, ethnic, and sexual identities from British Pakistani men who identify as Muslim and gay. *British Journal of Social Psychology, 49*(4), 849–870. https://doi.org/10.1348/014466609X485025

Jaspal, R., & Cinnirella, M. (2012). Identity processes, threat, and interpersonal relations: Accounts from British Muslim gay men. *Journal of Homosexuality, 59*(2), 215–240. https://doi.org/10.1080/00918369.2012.638551

Jaspal, R., & Cinnirella, M. (2014). Hyper-affiliation to the religious ingroup among British Pakistani Muslim gay men. *Journal of Community and Applied Social Psychology, 24*(4), 265–277. https://doi.org/10.1002/casp.2163

Jaspal, R., & Lopes, B. (2025a). Breadcrumbing by a dating partner, perceived social support, and paranoia. *Journal of Aggression, Maltreatment & Abuse*. https://doi.org/10.1080/10926771.2025.2555567

Jaspal, R., & Lopes, B. (2025b). Vulnerability to "breadcrumbing" in a sample of adults in the United Kingdom: A cross-sectional survey study. *Psychology International, 7*(3), 71. https://doi.org/10.3390/psycholint7030071

Kroger, J., Martinussen, M., & Marcia, J. E. (2010). Identity status change during adolescence and young adulthood: A meta-analysis. *Journal of Adolescence, 33*(5), 683–698. https://doi.org/10.1016/j.adolescence.2009.11.002

LaSala, M. C. (2000). Lesbians, gay men, and their parents: Family therapy for the coming-out crisis. *Family Process, 39*(1), 67–81. https://doi.org/10.1111/j.1545-5300.2000.39108.x

Markowe, L. A. (1996). *Redefining the self: Coming out as a lesbian*. Polity.

Markowe, L. A. (2002). Young lesbians: Coming out into the future. *Lesbian and Gay Psychology Review, 3*(1), 11–18. https://doi.org/10.53841/bpslg.2002.3.1.11

Matthews, C. H., & Salazar, C. F. (2012). An integrative, empowerment model for helping lesbian, gay, and bisexual youth negotiate the coming-out process. *Journal of LGBT Issues in Counseling, 6*(2), 96–117. https://doi.org/10.1080/15538605.2012.678176

Morrow, D. F. (2004). Social work practice with gay, lesbian, bisexual, and transgender adolescents. *Families in Society, 85*(1), 91–99. https://doi.org/10.1606/1044-3894.246

Orne, J. (2011). 'You will always have to "out" yourself': Reconsidering coming out through strategic outness. *Sexualities, 14*(6), 681–703. https://doi.org/10.1177/1363460711420462

Robins, R. W., Tracy, J. L., Trzesniewski, K., Potter, J., & Gosling, S. D. (2001). Personality correlates of self-esteem. *Journal of Research in Personality, 35*(4), 463–482. https://doi.org/10.1006/jrpe.2001.2324

Ryan, W. S., Legate, N., & Weinstein, N. (2015). Coming out as lesbian, gay, or bisexual: The lasting impact of initial disclosure experiences. *Self and Identity, 14*(5), 549–569. https://doi.org/10.1080/15298868.2015.1029516

Saltzburg, S. (2009). Parents' experience of feeling socially supported as adolescents come out as lesbian and gay: A phenomenological study. *Journal of Family Social Work, 12*(4), 340–358. https://doi.org/10.1080/10522150903261932

Savin-Williams, R. C. (2005). *The new gay teenager*. Harvard University Press. https://doi.org/10.4159/9780674043138

Index

R. Jaspal, *The Psychology of Coming Out*,
https://doi.org/10.1007/978-3-032-02599-9

The manufacturer's authorised representative in the EU is Springer Nature Customer Service Centre GmbH, Europaplatz 3, 69115 Heidelberg, Germany. If you have any concerns regarding our products, please contact ProductSafety@springernature.com

Printed and bound by CPI Group (UK) Ltd, Croydon, CR0 4YY
01/10/2026
02225854-0011